HELD BY THE

LAND

WA CH'ÍCH'ISTWAY
TA TEMÍXW

HELD BY THE
LAND

A Guide to Indigenous Plants for Wellness

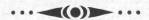

WA CH'ÍCH'ISTWAY TA TEMÍXW:
SPÉṄEM TXWNAṀ TA HA7LH SḴWÁLWEN

Leigh Joseph

wellfleet
press

First published in 2023 by Wellfleet Press, an imprint of The Quarto Group,
142 West 36th Street, 4th Floor, New York, NY 10018, USA
T (212) 779-4972 F (212) 779-6058 www.Quarto.com

Wellfleet titles are also available at discount for retail, wholesale, promotional, and bulk purchase. For details, contact the Special Sales Manager by email at specialsales@quarto.com or by mail at The Quarto Group, Attn: Special Sales Manager, 100 Cummings Center Suite 265D, Beverly, MA 01915 USA.

10 9 8 7 6 5 4 3

ISBN: 978-1-57715-294-1

Library of Congress Control Number: 2022943322

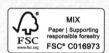

Group Publisher: Rage Kindelsperger
Creative Director: Laura Drew
Senior Art Director: Marisa Kwek
Managing Editor: Cara Donaldson
Editors: Katharine Moore and Elizabeth You
Cover Design: Marisa Kwek
Cover Illustration and Spot Art on the following pages by Sarah Jim: 2, 7, 8, 18-19, 20 *excluding Labrador Tea*, 30, 40 *excluding Plantain*, 50 *excluding Wapato*, 60 *excluding Saskatoon Berries*, 74, 92, 132, 160
Interior Art on the following pages by Ocean Hyland: 6, 21, 26, 29, 33, 37, 41, 44, 49, 53, 55, 57, 62, 65, 66, 69, 76, 78 *top left & right*, 80 *left*, 82, 86, 88, 90, 94 *left*, 96 *right*, 98 *left*, 102 *left*, 106 *left*, 108, 110, 114 *left*, 116, 118 *left*, 120 *right*, 122 *left*, 126 *left*, 128 *right*, 130 *left*, 134 *left*, 136, 138, 140, 144, 146 *left*, 148, 150, 152 *top*, 154 *top left*, 156 *right*, 158 *left*, 162, 164, 166 *left*, 168
Interior Art on the following pages by Marisa Kwek: 13, 16, 31, 35, 47, 51, 61, 70-71, 78 *base*, 80 *center & right*, 84, 94 *right*, 96 *left*, 98 *right*, 100 *base*, 102 *right*, 104, 106 *right*, 112, 114 *right*, 118 *right*, 120 *left*, 122 *right*, 124, 126 *right*, 128 *left*, 130 *right*, 134 *right*, 142, 146 *right*, 152 *base*, 154 *right & base*, 156 *left*, 158 *right*, 166 *right*
Interior Art on the following pages by Fernanda Alatorre: 39, 176
Interior Layout: Danielle Smith-Boldt

Printed in China

For my children, Ava and Jake.

CONTENTS

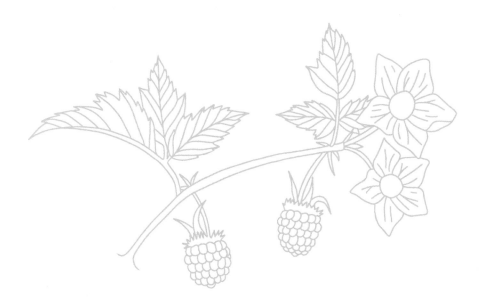

70 *Plant Profiles & Recipes*

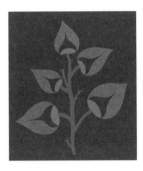 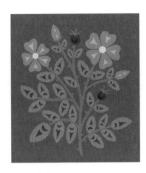 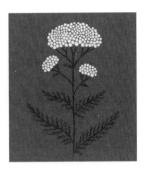 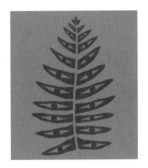

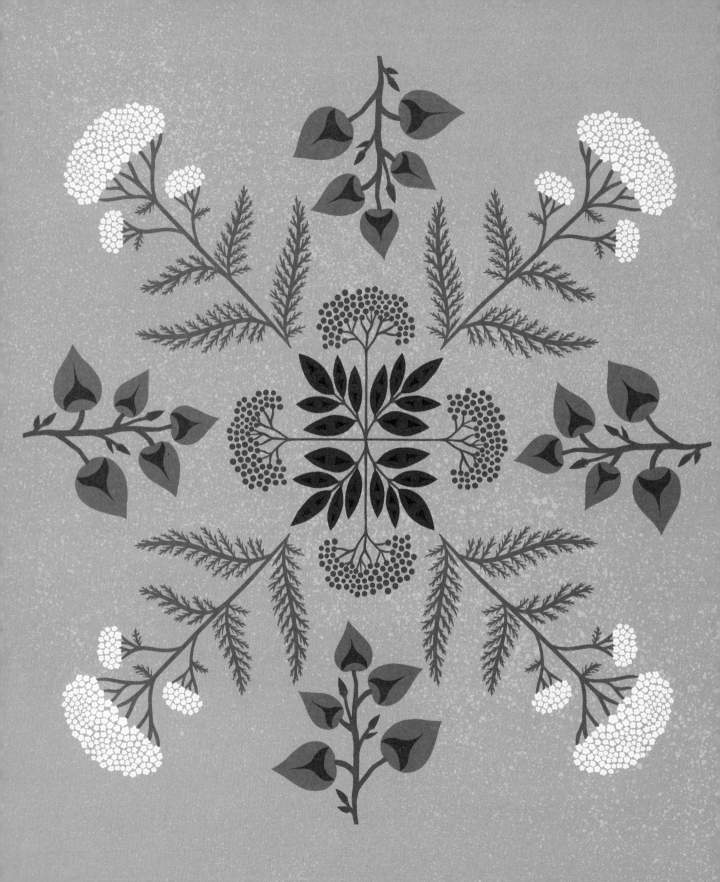

INTRODUCTION

∙∙∙◄●►∙∙∙

While I write this introduction, the season in the Pacific Northwest is turning toward spring. There are hints of new growth in the plants in my garden and on the trails around my home. Leaf buds are set, and soon the new shoots will start to grow up through the soil in the forests and estuaries in my home territory of Sḵwx̱wú7mesh (Squamish, British Columbia, Canada). As I have learned more about plants and their life cycles, I have developed a new sense of timing that is based on botanical seasonality. I look forward to the return of early-spring plant foods and medicines and the harvesting time spent on the land with family.

I am an Indigenous ethnobotanist, woman, mother, and entrepreneur. All the work I do in my life has been guided by plants. It has been through rebuilding my cultural relationships with the land, learning about plants, and reconnecting with them, that I have found grounding and strength in my identity. I was compelled to write this book for my children and for my community, and to share my voice as a Sḵwx̱wú7mesh woman in the spaces of botany, beauty, and self-care. There is very little Indigenous representation in these spaces, and it is my hope that my children, my community, and other Indigenous communities utilize this book as a helpful tool for reconnecting to culturally important plants. For non-Indigenous readers, I hope that this book resonates with your love of plants and the land and supports you in further developing your lived experiences and knowledge of what it means to you to be in respectful relationships with plants.

This book is meant to be an intersection between my lived experience as an Indigenous woman, my training in Western science, and my cultural journey toward identity. Part narrative, part botanical field guide, and part recipe book, it is a guide you can carry in a backpack or harvest basket, place on your kitchen shelf, or keep out on a table for quick reference. I intend this book to be a helpful companion and to support cultivating respectful and reciprocal ways of being in relationship with place and with plants.

This book covers plant species primarily found in the Pacific Northwest regions of North America. I have focused on plant species that I am most familiar with, but many of these plants have other species or closely related plants that span much farther geographically. The plants included in this book are not an exhaustive or complete list of all the culturally important plants that are found in this region. Instead, I have chosen plants that have a cultural history in my home territory of Sḵwx̱wú7mesh across a range of foods, medicines, and materials. I write this book from my Sḵwx̱wú7mesh perspective as I cannot speak for any other Indigenous Peoples or communities. I want to emphasize that Sḵwx̱wú7mesh is one of hundreds of diverse Indigenous communities in North America. It is my hope that sharing my perspectives on plants as an Indigenous woman will provide a lens for being in relationship with plants that resonates with Indigenous and non-Indigenous readers alike.

 ## About the Title

Held by the Land was one of many title options. This one rang true. What does it mean to be held? To me this means being seen, recognized, supported, allowed just to be. Being held also means being offered what you may need in a particular time, whether that be space, nourishment, health, connection, challenge, or reflection. The land can hold us, and our needs, as humans on this earth.

How does the land hold someone?

Through my work as an ethnobotanist, I have spent time listening to elders share stories of spending whole seasons and years on the land together with loved ones, working hard, being solitary, absorbing their natural surroundings, and actively being a part of the natural world. There were recurrent themes that I noticed—feelings of deep safety, contentment, strength, and good health. When I think about the times in my life where I have felt the most at ease, the surest about myself, the most connected, they were the times that I have spent on the land—out harvesting, planting, sharing a meal with my family on a big stump in the middle of a spring forest, my children nibbling on thimbleberry and salmonberry shoots. These moments that make up the highlights of my life were all supported by the land and leave me feeling held. I invite readers to take a moment to close your eyes. Think and feel your way into a meaningful and relaxing memory of time spent on the land. What season was it? Who was there with you? What sounds were around you? What plants were there? I believe we all share these moments in our lives where we catch a glimpse of the ongoing relationship we are in with the natural world. With relationship comes responsibilities as well. What do we offer back to the land, a presence that offers so much to us?

 ## Land-Based Wellness

Wellness is a very commonly used term in the English language. It often conveys practices connected to physical health and can extend in some cases to include mental, emotional, and spiritual health. I would like to bring another lens to that concept. While its focus is often on the individual, for the purposes of this book I wish to extend the concept of wellness to the interrelationships we experience with the natural world and with community, and what this means for our greater responsibilities and purpose as individuals sharing the earth together. The concept of community care can also be extended to the concept of wellness, and the definition of community can be extended to include our non-human kin, meaning *all* the non-human life that inhabits this planet. Along the way, we humans

Language

Language is intricately woven into identity and connection to place. Indigenous languages have undergone extensive impacts since the onset of colonization. There are many current, community-based language revitalization efforts happening in Indigenous communities across what is now known as North America. I chose to incorporate Sḵwx̱wú7mesh language throughout this book to honor the importance of language and the revitalization efforts taking place, and as a way to build new connections with plants from a Sḵwx̱wú7mesh perspective. I have included phonetic pronunciations (throughout this book as well as on page 177) so that you the reader can join in breathing new life into the Sḵwx̱wú7mesh language. When you say these words, I invite you to reflect on the hundreds of diverse Indigenous languages and dialects that exist across North America.

have elevated ourselves, in our minds and in the ways we live, over much of the other life on the planet. I propose that part of wellness in the context of this book is reexamining, rebuilding awareness of, and upholding our side of the relationships we build with the natural world. It also involves recognizing that our intentions and actions do hold meaning and can make a difference, and that no matter where we live or who we are, we are all supported by the land. When we uphold our side of this relationship, we also contribute to our own wellness, in addition to the wellness of our families and communities.

Plants as Relatives

When I teach in my capacity as an ethnobotanist, whether it is to postsecondary science students, elementary school children, or to Indigenous communities, I start by sharing how plants are considered relatives in a Sḵwx̱wú7mesh context. This belief in plants as relations frames the entire relationship with culturally important plants and the ecological habitats in which they grow. I explore what it means to be in relationship. How do dynamics shift when we are in relationship? What do respectful and reciprocal relationships look like? This shift in perception leads to a shift in values and in responsibility. Suddenly, if we are engaged in a relationship, we carry a responsibility to uphold our side of that relationship in meaningful ways.

For example, if I look out at a standing x̱ápay̓ay (western red cedar), and I see this as an economically important and valuable tree that can make money, that will lead me down a certain path of thinking and valuing the tree. Or I could look at that same tree as my relative and consider the needs of that tree, what I can do to care for the tree and its habitat, and the gifts it may offer me in exchange. These are two very different perceptions of the tree and its habitat. There is a teaching in Sḵwx̱wú7mesh culture that when you set out to harvest sléwéy (slaw-eye), or the inner bark of the x̱ápay̓ay, if you don't prepare yourself properly to offer an introduction and a thank you to the tree, if you intend to take too much bark from one tree, or if you harvest from a tree that has been previously harvested from, that tree will choose not to give much of its bark to you as a gift. The inner bark is an incredible material for weaving clothing, hats, basketry, and rope, along with other cultural and ceremonial applications. When you harvest the bark, you hope for a long, straight pull that can then be separated from the outer bark, cut into strips, and cured for up to two years (or until the sap dries up). It can then be utilized to create beautiful works of art. The bark is a gift, and it is one that relies on respect and reciprocity on the part of the harvester and the stewards of the land that the tree grows on.

What comes to mind when we think of relationships and the responsibilities we carry to uphold our side of the relationship with plants and the land? It is essential to understand the impacts on plants and the land and the related cultural knowledge and practices to rebuild respectful relationships. For me, the first things I think of are: How can I act to support this botanical relative? How have past or ongoing impacts shaped access to this plant? What can I do to uphold my responsibility to this plant? Sometimes this last question may lead to actions such as replanting parts of a plant, planting new plants in the place of the one you are harvesting, not harvesting at all, or taking only part of a living plant and leaving the rest in place. These actions will depend on the reproduction strategies and life cycles of the plant relative in question.

 ## Cautions, Warnings, and Responsibilities

Before you begin harvesting plants, there are some very important safety and ethical concerns. The following is a list of some of those key considerations. I invite you to add to this list depending on other possible risks (such as wildlife, terrain, climate, or others) in the regions where you live.

Poisonous Plants
Plants defend themselves creatively. One effective way is to produce compounds that can be poisonous to us humans or to other animals, including insects. You must familiarize yourself not only with the plants you wish to harvest but also with other plants that could be confused with your target

Harvesting

The term "harvest," in the context of this book, refers to taking material from plants that are either growing wild or planted in a garden setting. Wild harvesting from an Indigenous perspective is a practice that is embedded within a fabric of cultural knowledge, sustainable plant management, and ethical relationships. I encourage you as a reader to consider how you can build sustainable and respectful relationships with plants before harvesting, and to always consider growing your own native plants for use as food, medicine, or material.

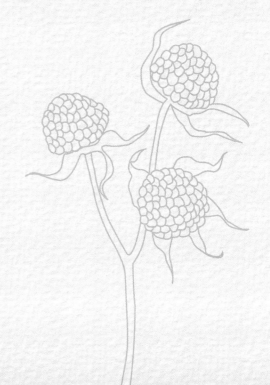

plant—especially if the look-alike plant could be poisonous. Another teaching that has been shared with me is that often the plants we utilize as medicines can become poisonous or inedible if we don't know how to prepare them properly. This may be in the timing of the harvest, as some plants change throughout their growing season and become inedible. It may be in the concentration of the medicine; some plant medicines will become too concentrated to ingest safely if you do not know how to prepare them properly.

This could be in the part of the plant you harvest; some plants have only certain parts that are safe to ingest, while other adjacent parts are poisonous or inedible. There may be contraindications for use of certain plant foods or medicines with prescription medications. This can be a tricky one to get clear answers on due to lack of extensive research on the topic; you will need to speak with your healthcare provider and (if applicable) the cultural knowledge holder you might be working with.

Native Plants and Native Plant Nurseries

Native plants are ones that grow naturally in a region, having evolved over thousands of years and developed symbiotic relationships with their surroundings. A non-native plant is one that does not grow naturally in a region. An introduced plant species is one that has been brought to a new region through human activities, either intentionally or unintentionally. An invasive plant species is one that is non-native, introduced, and becomes very competitive in its new environment, overtaking habitat that would otherwise be inhabited by native plant species.

Native plants offer nutritional diversity and a myriad of other benefits to non-human life, such as breeding habitat, food, and nesting areas.

Indigenous Peoples have resided alongside native plants for thousands of years and have developed deep interrelationships with them. Native plant nurseries specialize in carrying only plants native to their region, and engage in activities such as seed saving and propagating culturally important plants for their region as well. These nurseries are wonderful places to purchase native plants without putting pressure on wild plant populations. This is particularly important from a cultural standpoint, as many Indigenous Peoples and communities still have barriers to accessing culturally important plants. Overharvesting is also a concern, with rising interest in wildcrafting and foraging for native plants.

Sustainable Harvesting vs. Overharvesting

One of the best ways to avoid overharvesting is to purchase plants from a native plant nursery and grow them yourself. Considering what impacts your harvest will have on an ecosystem is critical. Thinking about the other species that rely on the plants will hopefully give us pause to think about how to ensure we are not taking too much ourselves.

Some plants could be endangered, sacred, or at risk of overharvesting. Familiarizing yourself with plant population monitoring and asking local Indigenous communities in your region will help you to avoid harvesting plants that fall into these categories.

Doing research and understanding the cultural history and present-day cultural use of an area is foundational to being respectful and ensuring you are not harvesting at sacred or culturally sensitive sites.

Contaminated Sites

Knowing the history of the sites where you harvest is important to understanding any contamination risks that might not be visually apparent. As a basic rule, do not harvest under powerlines or along railroad tracks or busy roads, as these are areas where chemicals may be sprayed on the plants. However, soil contamination from past industrial activity will only be evident if you research the history of the site.

When Not to Harvest

Sometimes it is just not appropriate to harvest. If you know a plant is endangered or sacred to a culture other than your own, don't harvest it. If you can see the plant is scarce in an area or the area has already been harvested from, don't harvest. If the harvest site is unsafe for some reason—contamination, wildlife, treacherous terrain—don't harvest.

Wildlife

When you go out onto the land, you are entering into the home of non-human life. Here in the Pacific Northwest, that may mean you could cross paths with a black bear or grizzly, a cougar or coyote. It is important to be educated and prepared for these encounters. This may mean harvesting in less-remote locations, going with a group, bringing some safety items (such as bear spray, a cell or satellite phone, and a first aid kit), and sharing a trip plan with someone at home.

Climate

Our climate is quite temperate in the Pacific Northwest, but you can get into more extreme weather and climate in high alpine or desert ecosystems. Rainfall and snow are both considerations depending on the season, terrain, or altitude. Most sea-level harvesting will not have extreme climate considerations, but if you are in areas within the northern regions of the Pacific Northwest, it is a good idea to ensure you are not at risk of avalanches, extreme cold, or other significant weather events.

General Safety and Planning

When you are planning to go out harvesting, it is always a good idea to go through the following checklist:

1 Are you one hundred percent confident in the identification of the plant you are planning to harvest?

2 Have you packed all the tools you will need for the harvest? This may include: a basket, clippers, gloves, long-sleeved shirts and pants, plant field guides (this book along with your favorite plant field book), a knife, sun hat and sunscreen, or more.

3 Are you going out with someone? Or have you let someone know where you are going and when you plan to return?

4 Have you checked the weather and planned accordingly? This is more important if traveling to remote areas.

5 Do you have a safety plan in place for encountering wildlife in your region?

Intergenerational Healing and Learning

When I became a mother, I was given a new lens to look at the world. One of love, responsibility, and strength. I wanted to provide opportunities for my children to fill in some of the gaps that I experienced in my life due to the impacts of colonization and intergenerational trauma on my family. My path to cultural reconnection through rebuilding relationships with plants and the land has become a path that my children follow as well. They do this in their own ways, and the experiences of being on the land together will settle into their lived memories in unique ways from my own. But I know in my heart that the days we spend together on the land, laughing, talking, nourishing ourselves, and quietly being, will all build a foundation within them to return to throughout their lives. That foundation is knowing that they belong. They are held. On the land. On Sḵwx̱wú7mesh temíxw, or Squamish lands.

How to Use This Book

This book holds a wealth of information for the plant lovers out there. The first section offers storytelling and reflections, as well as teachings and practices for developing respectful and reciprocal relationships with plants and with the lands where you live. There are teachings embedded within the opening chapters that have been shared with me by knowledge holders in my community and other Indigenous communities. I weave these cultural teachings together with my background as a botanist, as well as with my personal experiences working with plants. The second section of the book is part field guide and part recipe book for a selection of forty-four culturally important plants from the Pacific Northwest. Though the book does not comprehensively cover all the plants you will find in this region, you will get acquainted with some of the most iconic plant foods, medicines, and materials from the Pacific Northwest. Further to this, many close relatives of the plants included in this book extend into other areas of North America as well. It is my intention that this book facilitates hands-on and experiential learning with plants in ways that uphold our responsibilities to plants, to the land, and to future generations. Every action we take and every decision we make can be one that supports our environment and envisions a future for our great-great-grandchildren that is grounded in healthy ecosystems and access to the beautiful botanical gifts that these lands offer.

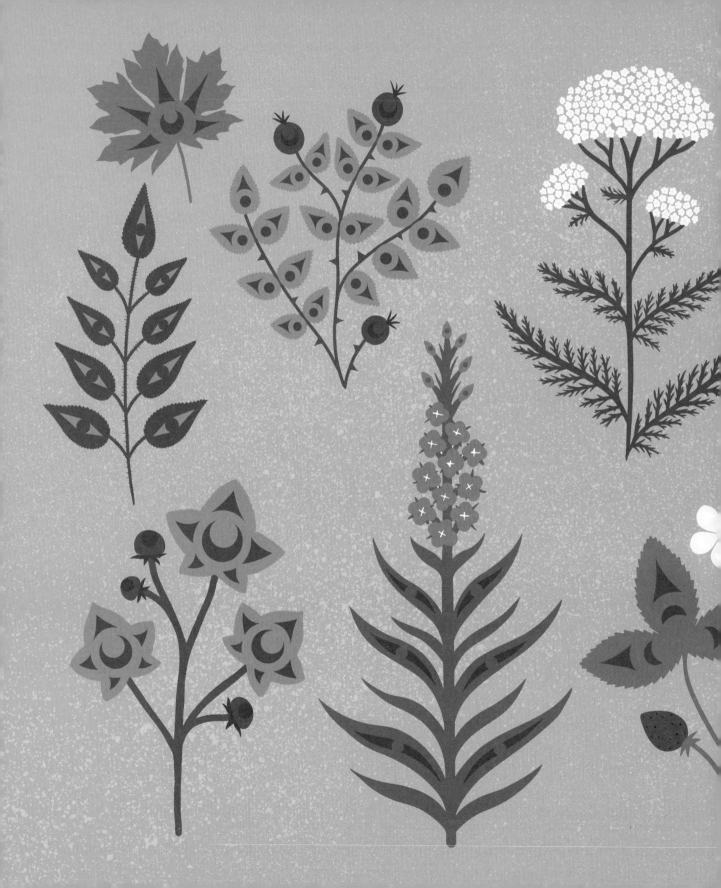

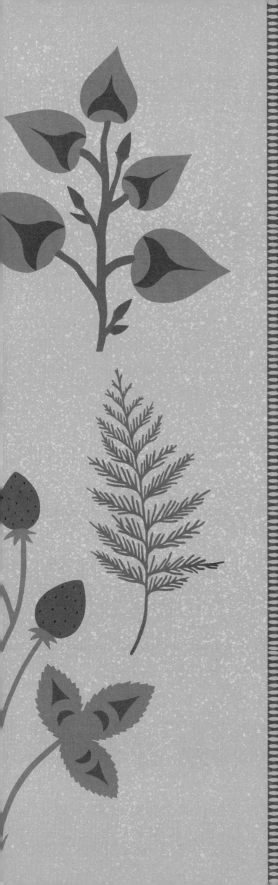

REFLECTIONS
*on Indigenous
Plant Knowledge
& Building
Relationships*

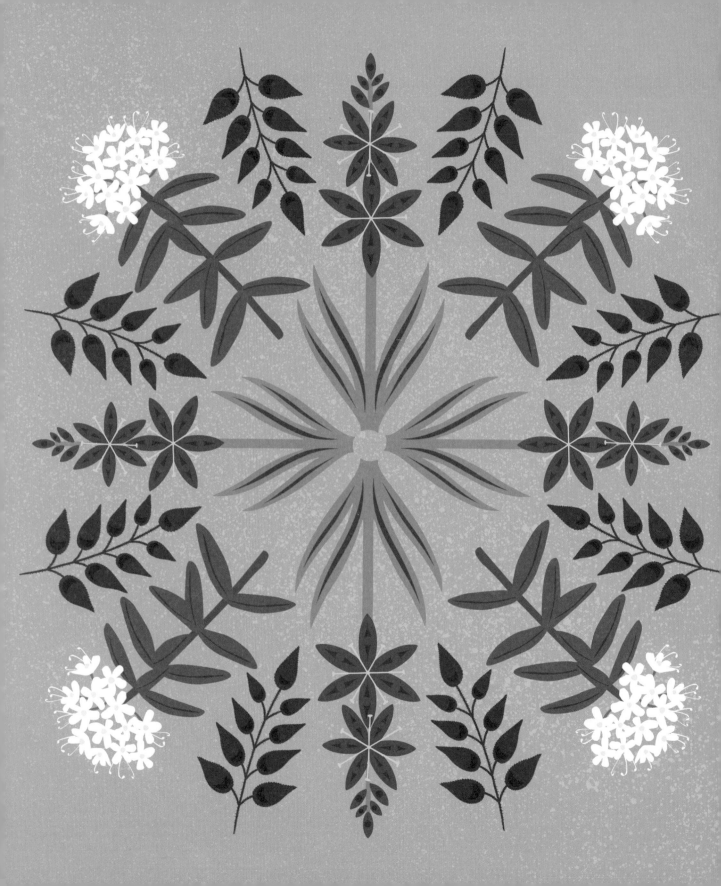

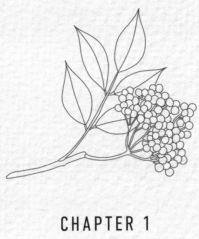

CHAPTER 1

Building Botanical Relationships

I remember as a small child feeling the most at ease close to home, solitary, outside in our front garden. My mom planted cosmos, yellow marguerites, and dahlias. I spent hours playing in the dirt, building tiny towns, weaving stories, imagining life in among the stems and leaves along my earthy playground. I recall the smell of the asphalt in the summer when the hose would soak it and I'd use dry leaves to rescue ants from the water rivulets. That brought me a great sense of contentment: to know that I had saved the lives of dozens of ants, all in a day's work and play.

My father, skwatatxwamkin siýam (skw-ah-ta-t-xw-am-kin see-am), Chief Floyd Barry Joseph, is a Coast Salish artist and carver. He started carving at age nine to help contribute to his family's income and has been creating artwork ever since. The smell of red cedar shavings defined my childhood. I spent hours watching him, back curved, leaning over a block of x̱payᵃ (red cedar) wood, helping the shape that he saw in it emerge into the world.

He sees the beauty and stories that are embedded in every standing x̱ápay̓ay (western red cedar) and each precious plank, block, and log that comes from this sacred tree. My dad often had a large carving or totem pole up on blocks in our front driveway. So, when I played outside, we would often be together but in our own worlds—creating and connecting to what it meant to be Sḵwx̱wú7mesh (Squamish) in our own ways from our little front yard in the area now known as Victoria, British Columbia (also known as BC). I didn't know it, but the pathway to my identity was being formed back then on those long, easy afternoons. Sitting in the garden, feeling the wind on my face, the sun on my back. Smelling the warm scent of cedar, hearing the chisel and sandpaper doing their work. Joni Mitchell drifting outside the house as my mom was inside creating the warmth and love that filled my childhood.

My mom is of English and Sephardic Jewish ancestry. She is a writer, a baker, and a poet through and through. She is openhearted and openminded, and so very supportive of the ones she loves. From a young age I remember her creating opportunities for connection to our Sḵwx̱wú7mesh ancestry. She has explained to me that she also found belonging, family, and support through marrying into my dad's Sḵwx̱wú7mesh family. I was an only child for the first five years of my life, and I recall visiting elders in the Sḵwx̱wú7mesh, Líl̓wat, W̱SÁNEĆ, Tseshaht, and Snuneymuxw territories with my parents. I recall feeling safe and comfortable sitting on the soft couches in these elders' living rooms. Sharing meals at the small kitchen tables covered in clear plastic. Smelling coffee and woodsmoke. Hearing the gentle and strong sounds of Indigenous languages being spoken, and the contagious laughter that inevitably would erupt at some point. I recall feeling the ease that comes with being in an environment where you know you're held in love and respect, without judgment or expectation. I was also quiet and pretty shy as a kid, so that helped me to be an observer. I was taking in connection and relationship and what it means to follow the cultural teachings of sitting with one's elders. I still draw on these experiences today when I'm sitting and learning from elders in the work I do with renewing cultural knowledge and experiences with plants.

A Rose by Any Other Name

When I was in high school, I was never considered a science student. It was clearly communicated that I should stay within the arts. I was intimidated by math, chemistry, and physics, but I loved biology. I remember that my Biology 12 class piqued my curiosity and interest for how life worked. It surprised me. Years later, when I decided to return to pursue postsecondary education, I heard about the field of ethnobotany: the study of the interrelationships between people and plants. I knew immediately this was what I wanted to study. I felt so excited by the prospect of being able to learn about plants from a cultural standpoint and work with Indigenous communities. I think I knew even then that this was a pathway home. Of the various fields through which ethnobotany can be studied, I decided I wanted to approach it scientifically. It was important to me to develop my understanding of the types of plant chemicals we utilize for medicine, the nutritional aspects of plant foods, and to finesse the proper identification of plants and the environments and ecosystems in which they flourish.

To pursue this path, I needed to upgrade all of my sciences to qualify for a university undergraduate double-major program in biology and environmental studies. My intimidation was matched by my enthusiasm. I *knew* I was on the right path even as I worked through chemistry, math, and statistics classes! I found the reaffirmation I needed in my first plant ecology field course. We learned about plant ecology and botanical field identification. We collected plants for herbarium pressings and for labs where we explored the structures of flowers under dissecting microscopes. I spent endless hours poring over my plant-name flashcards, learning the Latin binomial system of naming and categorizing plants. I learned the Latin name for western red cedar was *Thuja plicata*, salal was *Gaultheria shallon*, and that the salmonberry plant my dad taught me about was named *Rubus spectabilis*. I started to see the greenery around me in more detail, through a focused lens of wanting to identify my surroundings, to name them. I felt proud each time I could identify a plant along a trail somewhere.

I was learning a system of naming plants that had an old history in Western science. The Linnaean Taxonomy system, which was founded by Swedish naturalist Carl Linnaeus in the 1700s, organizes organisms into a two-part naming system: the first name indicating the genus, and the second part the species name. This system requires that the plant names be in Latin, and I've come to understand that often the names that were put on "newly discovered" plant species were the names of colonial figures.

Names are complicated and hold much meaning for and significance to identity and provenance. It did not occur to me at this stage in my educational journey to stop and critically think about this naming system. It was not until later that I began to consider what it might mean for names to have been imposed onto plants that had been in relationship with Indigenous Peoples long before recorded memory. I didn't know any of the Sḵwx̱wú7mesh plant names at that time. I was engrossed in calling the plants by these new names and enamored with how this naming system showed connections between closely related plant species and patterns displayed in particular plant families. It wasn't until I started my master's, when I received a digitization of an old audio recording of Sḵwx̱wú7mesh elders speaking the plant names in our Sḵwx̱wú7mesh sníchim, or Squamish language, that I started to feel the weight of imposition of names and the legacy of erasure, theft, and displacement that Latin names often carry with them. This was a turning point.

I remember sitting on the bus on my way to campus listening to the names spoken by members of my family that I had never met, pronounced in a foreign but deeply resonant language. I was so happy to hear plant names spoken in my ancestral language. I also felt sad that I hadn't had the opportunity to grow up learning these names in this language that was now endangered as a result of the colonial practice of eradicating Indigenous languages. I wanted to say the names correctly—to have them listed like a database in my brain, or perhaps embedded in my cells, where they would flow easily from my mouth and from my spirit. But the reality was I had never learned a word of our Sḵwx̱wú7mesh language. Both my grandparents attended residential school. They had their language beaten out of them. My father didn't grow up speaking or hearing much of the language and thus my siblings and I didn't either.

It's difficult to articulate the feeling of hearing the Sḵwx̱wú7mesh names spoken for the first time. Hearing the names shifted my entire framework. Suddenly there was an ancestral connection that resonated within me and grew into a desire to learn more, a purposeful drive to gather knowledge and then process it through my developing Indigenous lens—my unique Sḵwx̱wú7mesh lens. My maternal grandmother, Duna, (who I called Nani), loved Shakespeare. I recall her reciting lines from *Romeo and Juliet*: "What's in a name? That which we call a rose by any other name would smell as sweet." This is true. In fact, when I call rose by its Sḵwx̱wú7mesh name, ḵalḵáy, it smells even sweeter. The scent transports me to the generations before me of Sḵwx̱wú7mesh kin who have been in relationships with this plant from the time before memory.

Kwe7úpaý

Kwe7úpaý is the Squamish word for apple. My Nani gifted me an apple tree for my first birthday. She was pure magic to me. I associate her with the smell of fresh baking, the sound of CBC News playing in the background, singing coming from the kitchen, and her beautiful garden that stopped passersby daily. She was English and had moved from the Isle of Wight to North Vancouver with her first husband, John Dunn, a ship captain who died of tuberculosis shortly after they moved to Canada.

As for the apple tree, I of course don't recall receiving this early botanical gift. But over the years, I have heard the retelling of this story, and these recollections from family members have seamlessly formed into what feels like direct memory. The apple tree was planted in the backyard of our first home on Adanac Street in Lekwungen territory. I loved looking out and seeing my apple tree planted in the middle of the yard and watching it grow.

This was one of the first memories I have of being in relationship with a plant. I had a companion in that tree, another living being that was witnessing the world during my childhood years. A life to care for and observe, to sit with on my long afternoons in the garden. My family moved away from my childhood home when I was twelve, and my tree was too big to bring with us. I was heartbroken to leave my home and my tree.

I call this my tree, but I did not own it. Owning another living being was not the foundation of my childhood companionship with my apple tree. What mattered was having a presence so unlike myself but deeply connected to my story, my home. This early experience laid a path in me to view my natural surroundings, and the plants that live there, in a way that is rooted in kinship.

Indigenous Language as DNA

Indigenous language is the DNA of place-based relationship. It carries with it the unique accumulation of experiences, stories, wisdom, and interrelationships. By definition, DNA contains the instructions for how an organism develops, survives, and reproduces to carry on into the future. Just as DNA is the carrier of genetic information, language carries the blueprint for how to be in relationship with a particular place. Language has the power to completely alter how we view the world and the frameworks we apply to our families, communities, and natural environments.

Swé7u (s-weh-oh) means "to be named" in the Sḵwx̱wú7mesh language. I've been taught that when something is significant it is given a name. The word for April is tem tsá7tsḵay (tem ts-ah-ts-k-eye), which translates to "when salmonberry shoots are collected." May is tem yetwan (tem yet-wa-n) or "the time when the salmonberries ripen," and July is tem ḵw'élemew (tem kw-el-eh-mexw), meaning "the time when the blackberries ripen." August is tem t'áḵa7 (tem t-ah-ka), which translates to "when the salal berries are ripe."

There are place names as well, like T'ekw't'akw'emay (teh-kw-tah-kwem-eye), which translates to "place of many thimbleberry bushes." At the mouth of Evan's Creek, an ancestral village site, the name Ch'etch'at'iyay'em (ch-etch-at-y-eye-em) translates to "place of lots of devil's club" and corresponds with an ancestral harvesting site. The place-based cultural information that is embedded in language can teach us and guide us in how to reconnect to plants and the land. There are concepts in the Sḵwx̱wú7mesh language that do not translate to English, but when I as a Sḵwx̱wú7mesh woman learn them and speak them, I understand my existence in a new way. This creates a profound shift. Much practical knowledge of plants and place and history is encoded in Indigenous languages.

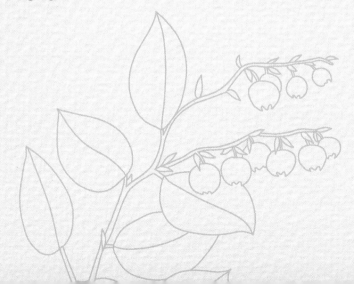

Impacts of Colonization on Botanical Knowledge

Since the time of European contact, Indigenous Peoples have needed to resource themselves with the strength and grounding that culture, the land, and community offer in navigating the impacts of colonization on culture, identity, ways of knowing, families, lands, plant knowledge and use, languages, and health and well-being. These impacts include loss of access to harvesting grounds, family time spent on the land, and healthy land-based foods and medicines. Adaptability, resilience, and reciprocity are important teachings that can be envisioned through plant/people interrelationships.

Indigenous Peoples across Canada have experienced a relatively recent and rapid shift away from their ancestral diets high in proteins, fats, oils, fiber, and fresh greens and berries, to contemporary diets high in sugars, saturated fats, and processed and refined foods, and low in fiber. The lack of healthy Indigenous foods is a sign of an "imposed poverty," as Anishinaabe scholar and community activist Leanne Betasamosake Simpson puts it. Prior to contact, the rich diversity of cultivated plant foods and medicines equated to a wealth that differs greatly from the contemporary definition of the word. As a result of the loss of access to Indigenous diet, there have been severe impacts on health in many Indigenous communities.

As an Indigenous ethnobotanist, the teachings for how to build respectful relationships with plants, along with the cultural belief of plants as relatives, have offered me guidance for how to heal from my own experiences with intergenerational trauma, as well as support the resurgence of plant-related knowledge and practices within Indigenous communities.

Indigenous Community Research

One of my academic mentors, Dr. Nancy Turner, helped me to integrate land-based learning experiences in Indigenous communities throughout the course of my university experience. Through her guidance, I participated in a program for Indigenous students where I was able to spend two six-week rotations working in Indigenous communities. The first rotation I spent working in the historic estuary root gardens in the area now known as Kingcome Inlet, home to the Musgamakw Dzawada'enuxw (musk-ka-ma zow-eh-dane-ook) First Nation who are part of the broader Kwakwaka'wakw people.

This experience was the first time I witnessed the remnants of historic estuary root gardens, called t'aki'lakw (ta-key-lack) in Kwak'wala. These gardens span the coast of the Pacific Northwest and were extensively cultivated to increase the productivity of key root vegetables. Remnants of these gardens are still present to the trained eye, but many of these extensive, historic gardens have been lost to development, industry, and urbanization. The t'aki'lakw in Kingcome is one of the most intact gardens that I've seen. You can still see the change in the density of rice root (*Fritillaria camschatcensis*), springbank clover (*Trifolium wormskioldii*), and pacific silverweed (*Argentina pacifica*), three of the culturally important root foods cultivated in these gardens.

The first time I dug up a rice root bulb in Kingcome it was the size of a potato—large enough to provide a substantial amount of starch to a meal. It was only after I started digging up the bulbs of rice root in the Sḵwx̱wú7mesh estuary that I saw how much smaller and densely packed they were, and I realized this is how rice root grows when it is untended. The traditional management of this species was to weed and till the surrounding soil and use a specialized digging stick—usually made from the high-tensile-strength wood of a yew tree (*Taxus brevifolia*) or ocean spray shrub (*Holodiscus discolor*)—to dig it up to harvest, and then replant some of the bulblets and the central corm of the bulb. The bulb of rice root looks like a ball of rice grain-like bulblets; each of these bulblets can grow into a new plant. As I explored more rice root in the Sḵwx̱wú7mesh estuary, it became clear to me that without the cultural relationship between plant and people in place, the rice root showed diminished productivity and density. With Indigenous weeding, tilling, and replanting practices, rice root was able to grow more successfully. The long-standing interrelationship between Indigenous Peoples and rice root led to an enhanced productivity of the plant and was supported through sustainable harvesting. When Europeans arrived in the country now known as Canada, they mistook the landscapes as being untouched and wasted, and used this misconception of *terra nullius* ("nobody's land") to justify the dispossession of Indigenous lands across North America.

This first chapter has explored the ways that I have built relationships with plants and the land from a cultural and personal context. Building personal relationships with the land and with plants is a rich process full of opportunities for observing and *feeling* how your natural surroundings support you and what you can offer in return. The next section will explore what teachings plants carry and what we can learn when we are more attuned to plants and the environments in which they are found growing. I encourage you as a reader to reflect on how you see building your own relationships with plants and the places that are special and important in your life.

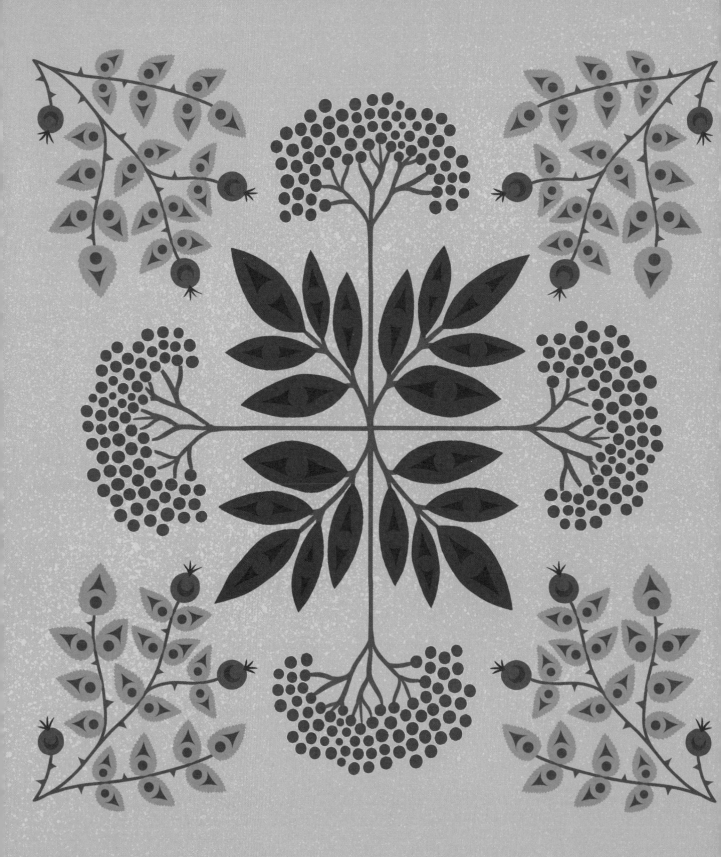

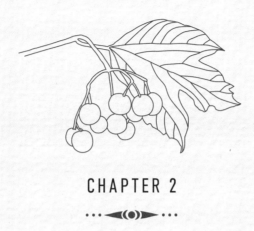

···◄(●)►···

Teachings from Plants

In Mary Siisip Geniusz's book *Plants Have So Much to Give Us, All We Have to Do Is Ask*, the author shares her Anishinaabe botanical teachings, offering another perspective on botany and what it means to build relationships with plants. This includes not only how to study or document or collect samples of plants, but how to be in relationship with plants and also with the lands on which they grow. I would also offer that plants have so much to *teach us* and all we need to do is *listen*. My aunt taught me that plants will communicate through dreams, visions, and visitations. She gently shared with me that while I was studying a Western scientific approach to learning about plants, there was also another path that I could walk concurrently that would open other aspects of working with plants . . . and that was to open myself to building relationships with, and being in relationship with, my botanical relatives.

I wish to share the following teachings from, and related to, plants that have been impactful in my life and in my community-based research work as an Indigenous botanist. The following teachings are ones that I continue to learn and integrate into my life to bring ongoing awareness and connectivity with my natural surroundings.

Tem' – Season | Following Seasonal Cycles

I have always tried to be aware of my surroundings, to pay attention to the changes in scent, in the quality of light, and in what plants are flowering. To feel the sun on my face and skin in all the various seasons: the cool chill of a spring morning that hints to warmer afternoons, the still heat of the summer, and the crisp transitions to fall.

I have also always noticed how I feel at different times in the year: how my mood and energy shifts, what I crave and wish to spend my time doing. Plants move their energy throughout their seasonal growth cycles and over the course of their life cycle, and rely on environmental changes in light, temperature, and moisture to signal when it is time to wake up and move into another part of their seasonal cycle. The region I live in is now known as the Pacific Northwest. This part of the world is characterized by a cool, wet climate, and landscapes blanketed with lush, temperate rainforests. During the shorter, colder winter months, plants gather their energy into their roots and wait for the signals of spring before they mobilize energy and nutrients toward seasonal growth. I love likening my seasonal cycles of life to those of my botanical teachers, taking time to renew in the colder, darker months so that when the springtime arrives I have the energy and vision to bring forth new growth. I believe creativity relies on these slow, reflective periods where we can integrate the seasons of long days, high activity, energy, and warmth.

Tímin – Strength | Building Resilience

Plants teach us about adaptability and resilience. Plants can thrive under certain levels and types of pressures. They can adjust to changes in their habitats and access to water and nutrients. Some can morph in shape and size to access favorable habitats or essential resources. Plants can store their seeds or bulbs under the ground until conditions are optimal for them to emerge from under the soil. One such plant that I often think of is spánanexw (camas). The purple flowers of camas once blanketed meadows that were maintained through Indigenous land-based knowledge, relationships, and practices, including fire management. The habitat for this plant has been severely impacted by development and industrialization, but the bulbs often still lie dormant under parks, fields, parking lots, and playgrounds—waiting until the relationship of fire and cultural management returns so they can burst forth from the earth. Cheryl Bryce, a friend of mine from Lekwungen, shared with me that when she has brought fire management back to areas of her traditional territory, camas has sprung back and thrived even after years of dormancy. Plants teach us about being connected and in relationship with place. They hint of a time when there were intensive systems of plant management and cultivation based on respectful relationships and the understanding that we are not dominant over plants, but instead in relationship with and often reliant on them.

 ## Slhílhkw'iws – To Be Connected | Interconnectivity

During my undergraduate studies, I took courses on the taxonomy, biochemistry, and cell biology of plants. Although I was fascinated to learn about the science of studying plants, I was also plagued by a feeling of unease. As I focused on particular cellular processes in plants and learned the nomenclature for how to speak about plants in a scientific way, I recalled concepts I had learned from my teachers and elders in my community of Skwxwú7mesh and other Indigenous communities I had worked with. These were teachings about connection: how ecosystems and the life growing in them are all connected, and that we as humans relying on the plants and other life in those ecosystems are also all connected. Contemplating the interconnectivity between all life created the foundation I needed to contextualize what I was learning in my academic setting and apply it to the culturally grounded way of viewing the natural world.

In her book *Finding the Mother Tree,* forest ecologist Suzanne Simard delves into the intricate interconnections that take place under the forest floor between tree roots and mycorrhizal fungi. Her groundbreaking research as a female scientist, but also as an individual who grew up in deep connection with forests and the natural world, challenged the hubris of the forest industry in the 1990s. When Simard started working in forestry it was mandated that entire tracts of forest be killed using harsh pesticides and herbicides, only to replace them with lucrative monocultures of high-value timber species. What forestry science didn't see at the time were the incredibly intricate interconnections between plants, soil, roots, trees, and fungi that a healthy and thriving forest ecosystem relies on. This strategy caused many problems due to the consequent loss of this interconnectivity and biodiversity. When I read about these unsustainable forestry practices that were, and are still in some cases, widely used within the Pacific Northwest, I considered the thousands of years of Indigenous cultural forest management and how this history brings another layer of human interconnectivity with forests— one that was overlooked by and absent from the forest industry, but centralizes living in relationship with the forest. We all benefit from recognizing that we, as humans, are interconnected with nature and not separate or above it.

Supporting Identity

I have had the gift of spending time with elders on the land and water in their traditional territories, and I have witnessed how their being in relationship with plants and the land directly supported their identity. These times have been formative to how I move in the world of research, teaching, entrepreneurship, parenting, and more. These elders *knew* their lands, plants, and waters. This often looked like having a compendium of memories and practical lived knowledge at their fingertips, a running map or chart of the territory in their minds, and a deep appreciation for the lands and plants of their homelands. I remember traveling by boat through an archipelago and harvesting edible seaweed with an elder, Kwaxsistalla, whose grandparents had hidden him in one of the bays among the maze of islets and larger islands when he was a child. They were hiding him from the Indian agents who at the time were stealing children from their homes and forcing them to attend residential schools.

As we whipped by shorelines that looked the same to me, Kwaxsistalla pointed out features without taking his eyes off the horizon ahead of us. I imagined a running chart in his mind, filled with the Kwak'wala place names that his ancestors laid across the land- and seascape. Directing us to stop at a rocky point on a small islet that looked the same as so many we had passed, he told me to climb up on the rock and lay out our harvested seaweed in square cakes. He said to stay up there and watch the cakes until one side felt drier and tacky; then I was to turn it over. I followed the instructions and noticed immediately that the seaweed cakes dried much faster on this rock than on the other rocks we had dried them on earlier in the day. I turned the seaweed cake and the other side dried even faster. As I waited, I looked out at the ocean and felt the wind on my face and the sun warming the rock below me. I noticed how the currents moved around the tip of the rock where it plunged into the sea, and I saw the profile of Kwaxsistalla as he waited patiently in the boat.

When I collected the dried seaweed cakes and headed back down to the boat, I learned that Kwaxsistalla had brought us to his grandmother's seaweed-drying place. Based on her deep knowledge of this archipelago, she had selected this exact spot because it had the right slope to the rock and the right exposure to winds and sun to dry the seaweed evenly and quickly. This moment has stayed with me as a poignant expression of the beauty and brilliance of place-based knowledge and how that knowledge carries with it story, context, and meaning that tie people to their ancestral territories in profound and enduring ways.

The Allure and Beauty of Plants

Plants hold ancient and ethereal allure. They have supported health, nourishment, spiritual awakening, and ceremony since time before memory. I remember being on a plant walk in a bog and learning that the ancient *Lycopodium* (club mosses) we were observing evolved some 410 million years ago, long before the time of the dinosaurs and the first humans. It humbled me to know that I was sitting in the presence of one of the most ancient vascular plants in the world.

And then to think about flowers! What a perfect balance of beauty and brilliant functional design. Based on fossil records, flowering plants are believed to date back to approximately 140 million years ago and to have diversified and specialized their strategies and design since their origin. Today there are close to 400,000 flowering plants identified in the world. The stunning diversity of flower shapes, colors, scents, nectars, and structures is an accumulation of changing relationships and coevolution between flowering plants and their pollinators and environments. When I read scientific papers on the coevolution of flowers and pollinators, I immediately think about the coevolution of Indigenous Peoples with botanical foods, medicines, and materials. Over time, Indigenous plant-management practices have also selected for certain characteristics and impacted the lineages of culturally important plants that provided nutrition, medicine, shelter, clothing, and so much more. There is rich oral history involving plants, and much lived Indigenous knowledge and experience about how to enhance their productivity through management techniques including prescribed burning, weeding, tilling, replanting, pruning, and more. These management techniques are an extension of plant/people relationships and often are woven together with ceremony and spiritual belief.

Relationship-Based Ecosystems

There are many examples of ecosystems that have been in relationship with Indigenous Peoples for thousands of years, and would be considered systems of management or cultivation. Forests are highly productive and important ecosystems for all Indigenous Peoples in North America. Many trees are culturally important, and other shrubs and herbaceous plants provide traditional foods and medicines. Though forests don't appear at first as productive food-growing areas for human use, there are areas of temperate forests that have been managed traditionally for millennia by Indigenous Peoples living in what is now known as North America.

Historically, forest gardens (also known as orchard gardens) were cultivated and managed areas of forest cleared of large conifers and planted with culturally important trees, shrubs, and plants. These forest gardens held, and still hold, a highly productive, concentrated biomass of culturally important plant foods. Temperate forest gardens in the Pacific Northwest are composed of an upper layer of mostly small fruit and nut trees, an understory of various berry species, and a forest floor of herbaceous plants that are nutritionally and medicinally important. Though there are variations depending on where the forest garden is located, these Indigenous managed food systems are characterized by species such as:

- hazelnut (*Corylus cornuta*)

- Pacific crab apple (*Malus fusca*)

- highbush cranberry (*Viburnum edule*)

- red elderberry (*Sambucus racemosa*)

- false Solomon's seal (*Maianthemum racemosum*)

- Nootka rose (*Rosa nutkana*)

- salmonberry (*Rubus spectabilis*)

- black hawthorn (*Crataegus douglasii*)

- Saskatoon berry (*Amelanchier alnifolia*)

- thimbleberry (*Rubus parviflorus*)

- wild raspberry (*Rubus idaeus*)

- black huckleberry (*Vaccinium membranaceum*)

Additionally, understory plants, including dense stands of Northern rice root (*Fritillaria camschatcensis*), stinging nettle (*Urtica dioica*), and fireweed (*Chamaenerion angustifolium*), grow along the edges where the gardens meet the unmanaged forest edge.

These food systems hold an incredible concentration of delicious and nutrient-dense plant foods. Furthermore, all these plant foods store well, making them important for supporting nutrition and energy through the winter months. These managed food systems persist today, some 150 years after tending to the gardens stopped due to impacts of settler colonialism and rapidly changing times. Some of the traditional management practices included pruning, coppicing, and transplanting trees and shrubs. These tree management practices, including intensive pruning and topping, are still evident in the shapes of the branches and enduringly easy access to crab apples from branches growing closer to the ground. The density of the aforementioned tree, shrub, and herbaceous plant species in forest clearings is a well-known indicator of old village sites. These include the extensive historical orchard gardens found at Robin Town, known as Dałk Gyilakyaw, in the Kitsumkalum Valley in Tsimshian territory.

In the early spring, the fresh green shoots of salmonberry, thimbleberry, and fireweed are eaten as delicious spring greens. The delicate outer green skin is peeled off and the juicy shoots are eaten raw or cooked. As the season progresses, the tender green shoots of stinging nettle come up and are ready for harvest as a nutrient-dense spring green, rich in iron, calcium, vitamins, and fiber. Following this time, multiple berry bushes go to flower and then progress to berries. The juicier berries such as salmonberries and raspberries historically were eaten fresh, whereas slightly less-juicy berries such as thimbleberries, salal, Saskatoon berries, and black huckleberries were dried into cakes or stored in airtight bentwood boxes submerged in water for use later in the season. In the late summer and fall, the fruit of hazelnut, crab apple, and rosehips ripen and are ready for harvest and storage for use through the winter. In the fall, the mature stalks of both stinging nettle and fireweed can be broken open to harvest the inner fibers; these were used to make twine for fishing lines and nets, and in some traditions added into mountain goat wool for weaving.

When you walk through a forest in winter, it is more difficult to see how the forest could provide a nutritious meal and vitamin-rich foods to maintain one's health. Thus, it was and is so important to have access to these culturally important, nutritious foods along with the expertise and knowledge for how to prepare and store them through the winter. These days we may use a canner, dehydrator, or freezer to prepare and store these foods. However, in pre-contact times, many of these foods would be dried into cakes or stored in water- or oil-filled bentwood boxes to be cherished and enjoyed through the winter months until the new, green growth of plant foods and medicines returned in the spring. Understanding the lifecycles of plants, how to optimize their habitats for growth and productivity, and when and how to harvest, process, and preserve foods, was and continues to be critical as more Indigenous communities reclaim plant knowledge and related practices to support their own land-based health and wellness practices.

Plants produce secondary compounds, which are chemical by-products of the plant's primary cellular processes, such as photosynthesis and cellular respiration. Secondary compounds are not essential to the plant's survival, but instead benefit the plant through actions like deterring insects and other animal life that would eat them, inhibiting bacteria, microbes, and fungi, or absorbing UV rays to protect leaves from being damaged by sunlight. These are the chemicals in plants that we humans have learned to utilize for medicines. I remember the feeling when I tried my first devil's club tea, a highly anti-inflammatory and immune-boosting plant medicine due to its secondary compounds. It was transformative. I am enamored with the beauty and brilliance of plants and the ways that people have learned to integrate them into health practices over thousands of years. There are also many nutritional values to plant foods that we will explore in the second part of this book. First, though, it is important to take time to consider and understand how to harvest plants sustainably and respectfully. Chapter 4, The Mindful Harvest, will offer a framework to do this, but please consider adding in your own layers of cultural or botanical knowledge and context.

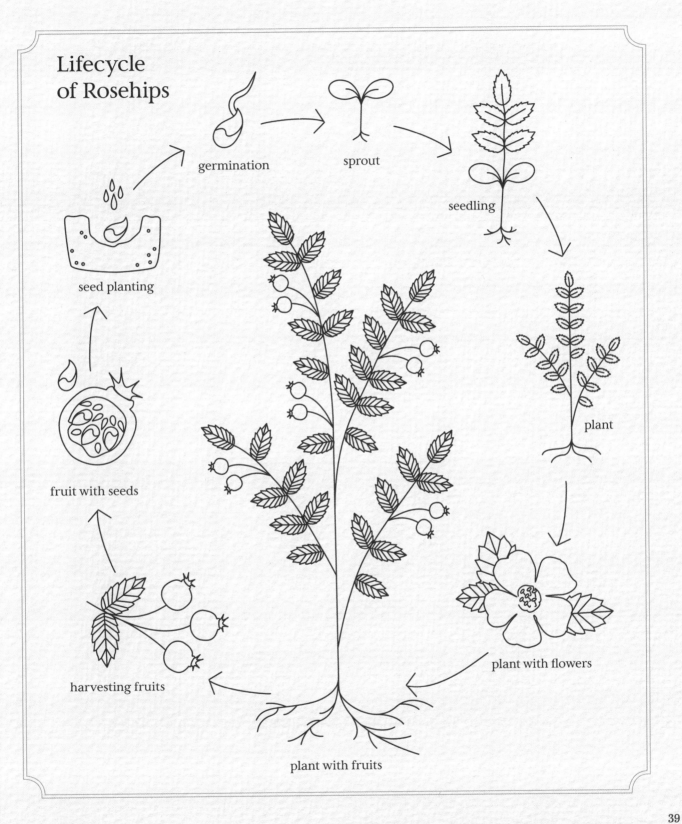

Lifecycle of Rosehips

germination

sprout

seedling

seed planting

plant

fruit with seeds

plant with flowers

harvesting fruits

plant with fruits

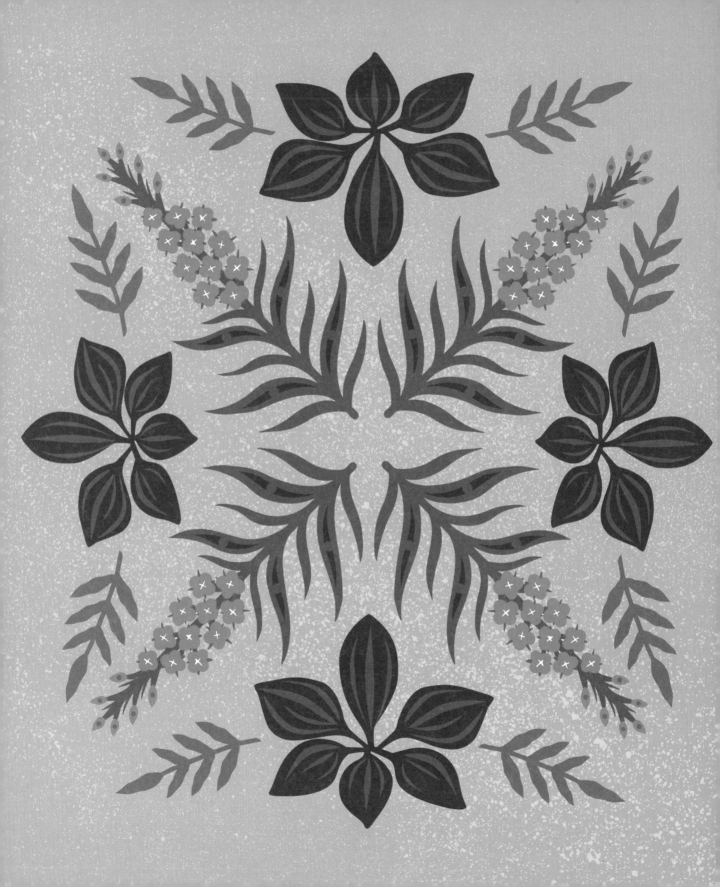

CHAPTER 3

Identifying Plants to Build Your Home Apothecary

Now that we have explored how to build respectful and reciprocal relationships with plants, we can look at building your own apothecary at home! Whether you are wild harvesting, growing in your garden, or purchasing plant ingredients from suppliers, there are some materials you will need to have on hand to help store dried plant ingredients, and some basic kitchen equipment that will help you process those ingredients.

First, it is important to ensure you have the tools to identify the plants you wish to harvest or grow. This first section will provide you with some tools and considerations for honing your plant identification skills.

Apothecary Wish List

MUST-HAVES:

Large jars to store dried plant materials: Darker glass may extend shelf life and potency by protecting from sunlight, moisture, and airflow.

Cheesecloth and/or fine-mesh strainer: You will be straining plant materials out of carrier oils. These items help ensure you don't leave plant matter in oils, as it can cause oils to spoil faster.

Measuring cup: You will want either glass or metal, as plastic can take on color or odor from certain plants. Having a range of sizes from 1–10 cups is nice, depending on the scale of the batches you are making.

Coffee grinder: A coffee grinder set aside only for plants is great for grinding them to make tea or other recipes.

Pestle and mortar: You will use these for grinding plant materials to blend into recipes.

Secateurs or scissors: Use the fine-tip models for clipping and processing plants.

PLANT-BASED CARRIER OILS:

A plant-based oil is one that is pressed from plant ingredients to produce an oil. A carrier oil is an oil infused with botanical ingredients, with the aim of extracting the benefits of the plant into a topical or ingestible oil. There are many beautiful carrier oils to choose from; I encourage you to do your own research, but I will share some of my favorites here. Just a note: if you are planning to infuse an oil for cooking or ingesting, make sure you find a food-grade oil. I like to opt for organic oils wherever possible, as these are generally made without harmful synthetic additives.

 Sunflower oil (*Helianthus annuus*) is rich in oleic acids and vitamins A, D, and E. Sunflower oil also has beneficial amounts of lecithin and unsaturated fatty acids, and is deeply nourishing and conditioning for the skin. This oil has a mild scent, is easily absorbed, and stores well under any condition—but avoid extreme heat and light, as these will lessen its shelf life.

 Jojoba oil (*Simmondsia chinensis*) is actually a liquid wax that closely resembles sebum (the oil in our skin), and is rich in vitamin E. Both properties promote a glowing complexion. The oil is bright and golden in color with a mild odor, and is highly regarded as a carrier oil because of its advanced stability and shelf life.

 Olive oil (*Olea europaea*) is one of the most universal oils, and is used for purposes including cosmetics, as a carrier oil, and for hair and skincare solutions. It is also great in cooking, and has a full-bodied flavor, nice olive-green color, and rich scent.

 Sweet almond oil (*Prunus dulcis*) is a fantastic carrier oil. It is light, quickly absorbed, has a subtle scent, and makes a superb addition to body-care products. People with nut allergies should avoid this oil.

 Grapeseed oil (*Vitis vinifera*) is an excellent oil to dress your favorite salads and other fine foods, and can be used for cosmetic products as well. It is often incorporated as a base oil for many creams and lotions, and as a general carrier oil. Grapeseed oil is especially useful for skin types that do not absorb oils well, as it does not leave a greasy feeling and absorbs well.

Plant Identification

Plants are all unique and have key features that will help you to identify them accurately with some practice. Knowing what part of the plant you are harvesting is also important. Whether you are harvesting leaf buds, leaves, flowers, roots, or bark will change how you approach the harvest. Observation is a big part of this learning process. This includes observing how the plant changes throughout the seasons and noticing what insect or animal life is also in relationship with this plant. The following sections will help you develop your plant identification skills.

Region and Ecosystem

As a high-level starting point, knowing in what region the plant you are interested in harvesting grows is important. Looking at this information can give you a sense of the distribution of the plant. If you are already familiar with the plant, learning more about what ecosystem(s) the plant is present in can help you start to predict areas where you will find that plant growing. This can aid in spreading out your harvesting activities across different areas or give you information for growing the plant in your garden. For example, if the plant likes to grow in well-drained soils, full shade, or sun, this will help you to decide where to plant it.

Timing

Paying attention to plants and your natural surroundings and how they change throughout the year can help in further understanding how or when to harvest. I keep a field journal to record the dates and places that I harvest in a season so I can refer to it for the timing of harvests and to make sure I visit different harvest areas season after season. My journal is full of pressed flowers and leaves and carries with it some of the soil from each harvest site.

Flowers

Flowers are a very helpful identification aid, but they are not present on the plant year-round in temperate regions, so knowing when to look for them can be helpful. Flowers come in a range of shapes, sizes, and colors, and knowing how to identify them is an important and enjoyable skill to develop. After all, who wouldn't want to spend time becoming more acquainted with flowers?

When setting out to identify flowers, you will pay attention to aspects such as color, shape (individual or clustered), size, number, and type of petals (separate or fused), and scent.

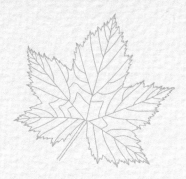

Leaves

Leaves are not always present in deciduous plant species, but they often remain on the plant longer than flowers. For leaf identification, you will pay attention to aspects such as leaf margin, leaf shape, the patterns of the veins in the leaf, thickness and texture, and, in some cases, scent.

Seeds

After the flower is pollinated, the seed will develop. This stage can take on many forms depending on the strategy for dispersing the seeds, which include wind, water, bursting open, being eaten, or attaching to animal fur, feathers, or clothing. The appearance of seeds will vary based on their dispersal strategy, but the seedpods or fruit that carry the seeds, for example, can be very helpful in plant identification. In some cases, it is the seed that you may be setting out to harvest or that can potentially be collected for planting or restoration purposes.

Bark

Trees and shrubs will have characteristics in their bark that can be helpful in identifying them. You will be looking at the color and texture, including whether the bark is smooth, rough, papery, has resin blisters, or other defining features. If you are harvesting the bark from a plant, timing is key. You can only access the inner bark of a plant when the sap is running in the springtime. This is the time when the plant mobilizes the stored energy and nutrients from its roots up into the aboveground parts of the plant to support new growth. It is at this time that the new inner-bark growth can be separated from the heartwood of the plant.

Roots

You will likely only see the roots of a plant if you are intending to harvest it or you're planting it out in the garden. If you are harvesting the root of a plant for food or medicine, it is a good trick to keep the aboveground plant parts attached to the root so you can be one hundred percent certain you have the right plant root. Roots can take various forms including taproots, bulbs, corms, rhizomes, and fibrous root systems.

Building Your Home Apothecary

Now that you have harvested your plants, you can begin to process and store them for later use. An apothecary is a collection of stored ingredients which can be extracted and combined for health benefits or to treat ailments. Historically, an apothecary could be equated with a modern-day pharmacy. This term, which has come back into general use, now can describe a collection of plant ingredients that carry topical and internal benefits. I do not go into detail about the medicinal applications of plants in this book, and there are many things to know before safely using plants medicinally. I would encourage you to do more research before making or ingesting medicinal preparations; these may include tinctures, decoctions, oxymels, capsules, and more. In this section, I will focus primarily on information for building an apothecary for everyday beauty and some food uses.

Plants for Beauty

Plants have supported beauty practices and rituals around the world for thousands of years, and have many beneficial properties when used topically. They can be incorporated into beauty and self-care rituals in a variety of ways, including facial steams, bath soaks, face masks, creams, balms, infused oils, and more.

Plants for Nutrition

Plants carry beneficial nutrients, vitamins, fiber, and more. Incorporating plants into your diet can be easy and fun with a bit of preparation and knowledge. Plants can be harvested and eaten fresh, dried for later use, or even powdered for ease in adding to soups, smoothies, and the like. Incorporating plants for nutrition can also support skin, hair, and nails from the inside out.

Plants for Medicine

Plants carry many beneficial compounds that support healing and ongoing good health. These may be integrated by eating the plant, drying it and making a tea blend, tincturing the plant, making an infused concentrate or syrup, and more. Plant medicines are powerful and must be treated with respect and care.

Plants for Material

Some plants provide materials for weaving, dyeing, carving, and other technologies. There is a long history and ongoing use of culturally important plant materials for technologies and artwork created by Indigenous Peoples.

Drying Your Plants

Unless you are planning to use fresh plant material, you will need a way to preserve the plant. One of the most common methods to preserve plants for later use is to dry them. There are some considerations for how to do this, including how delicate the plant is, how fast you want it to dry, and for what purpose you are drying the plant (i.e., tea, fruit leather, topical use).

Hanging to Dry

You will need:

- Clothesline you can hang somewhere cool and dry
- Elastics
- Clothespins
- Scissors

If you are harvesting plants that are leafy, have a stem, and can be easily bundled together, then hanging to dry is a great option. Setting up your drying area somewhere cool and dark will ensure the plants dry evenly and don't lose their potency as much as they would if they were dried in the sun. Use this technique if you wish to slowly dry plants. Harvest the plants on a dry day and, after the dew has dried up, follow these steps:

1 Bundle ten to fifteen stems together depending on the volume of the plant. You want the air to be able to dry all surfaces of the plant, so you don't want to bundle too many stems together.

2 Wrap an elastic around the bundle. If you use string the stems may shrink as they dry, and your bundle will fall on the ground.

3 Hang your plant bundles on the line using clothespins. Turn the plants regularly and check they are drying evenly.

4 Once fully dried, remove the plants and strip off the parts you wish to store for later use. For example, if you are saving the leaves, strip them off and compost the dried stem.

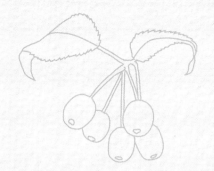

Sun Drying

You will need:
- Rack or clean area to dry plant materials on
- Sun and wind

In some cases, especially for food use with plants that are thicker or hold more moisture, it is appropriate to sun-dry them. Examples of this are seaweeds and wild berry fruit leather. The sun and wind can be very efficient at drying plant materials that would not dry hanging up.

Drying Racks or Baskets

You will need:
- Basket or drying rack with ample airflow
- Dark, cool place to gently dry plant materials
- Optional: a gentle fan

This is an ideal method for drying petals and delicate flowerheads; too much heat and direct sun will drain them of their color and fragrance, which you want to preserve as much as possible. You will need to shake the flowers a few times each day until they are dry to increase airflow and ensure all surfaces are drying.

Dehydrator

You will need:
- Dehydrator or oven
- Parchment paper

When drying heavier botanical materials such as bark, fruit, or wild berry fruit leathers, you can use either a dehydrator or an oven on low. If you will be processing a fair amount of plant material, it is worth investing in even a basic dehydrator; it is safer and the heat and drying are more consistent. In a pinch, you can dry plants in an oven set to 180–200°F (around 85–95°C) with the door propped open using a heat-safe item (such as a silicone mixing spoon).

Now that you have dried botanicals, you can find jars to store your treasured ingredients in until you are ready to use them.

Basic Oil Infusions

This is a general recipe for infusing dried botanicals into oils.

You will need:

- Double boiler
- Carrier oil of your choice (see page 42)
- Dried botanical material
- Glass quart (liter) jar
- Cheesecloth
- Fine-mesh strainer
- Rubber band

DOUBLE BOILER INFUSION METHOD

1 Pour water into the bottom pot of your double boiler; you don't want the bottom of your top pot to touch the water. Place the top pot in position and warm over medium heat.

2 Measure and pour the carrier oil into the top pot by the quart or liter.

3 Add ½–1 cup (66–140 g) of dried botanicals per liter of oil depending on how large the botanicals are. (For example, leaves will take up more space than rosehips.)

4 Allow the botanicals to gently warm in the oil for 2–4 hours. Be sure to check that the water has not evaporated in the lower pot! If it has, carefully remove the top pot with oven mitts, being careful not to spill hot oil, and add more water to the bottom pot. Then place it back on the heat with the top pot over the bottom pot.

5 Remove the double boiler from the heat. Let the oil cool to room temperature.

6 Prepare a clean, dry jar for strained oil. Line the strainer with cheesecloth.

7 Remove the top pot of the double boiler. Wipe the bottom of the pot with a dish towel to remove any condensation droplets so that they don't accidentally drop into your infused oil.

8 Carefully pour the oil into the jar, straining through the cheesecloth-lined strainer and being sure to remove all plant material from the oil. Repeat the straining step if necessary.

9 Compost the discarded plant material.

10 Store your infused oil somewhere cool and dry until you are ready to use the oil either as a body oil or as the base for a salve.

SUN INFUSION METHOD

1 For this method, follow the same ratios of ½–1 cup (66–140 g) of dry botanical material per quart (liter) of carrier oil.

2 Place the dry plant material in a large jar with the carrier oil. Place cheesecloth over the top of the jar and secure it with a rubber band.

3 Place the jar on a windowsill that gets direct sunlight and let it sit for 1–2 weeks to gently infuse into the carrier oil.

4 Follow steps 8–10 from the double boiler method.

 ## Powdering Botanicals

Whether you want to make a nutritional powder to add to oatmeal, soups, or smoothies, or to incorporate a favorite botanical into a clay facial mask or bath soak, many botanical ingredients (such as plants like stinging nettle, seaweed, or spruce tips, or flowers like rose or yarrow) are versatile when dried and powdered. For this step, you will need a coffee grinder or blender designated for powdering plants. I like to use a Vitamix® blender, as it is powerful and results in a fine powder. I purchased a second jug for my blender to use only for plant materials.

1 Clean your botanical ingredients to make sure there are no stray twigs or other unwanted materials.

2 Fill the blender half full with the dried botanicals. Blend on high with the lid securely on until the materials turn to a fine powder.

3 Turn the blender off and let any powder settle.

4 Take the lid off and pour powdered botanicals through a fine-mesh strainer if there are large particles left.

5 Pour the strained, powdered botanicals into a jar using a funnel and store somewhere dry and out of direct sunlight.

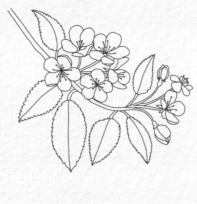

CHAPTER 4

···◄(●)►···

The Mindful Harvest

What is harvesting? When I use the word, I mean the act of going out on the land and taking plant foods, medicines, and materials from either wild or cultivated plant populations. Harvesting can look different depending on the plant. You may need clippers, a shovel, gloves, a basket.

What is a mindful harvest? It is a framework grounded in respect, reciprocity, and responsibility to plant relatives, and is foundational to being in good relationship with plants. Plants and the land have agency. They have their own spirits, names, interconnections, needs, and power. Being mindful with plants and with ourselves while observing, identifying, cultivating, and harvesting them is part of upholding our side of the relationships between people and plants.

Before I Harvest

My lived experience as an Indigenous woman, along with what my elders and cultural teachers have shared with me, has led me to ask myself questions before I set out to harvest. These questions come from a place of developing a humble self-awareness grounded in gratitude for the gifts of nature. They rely on an inherent understanding that I am relying on the generosity of the botanical relations that I am approaching, and that if I am not carrying myself in a good way, I will not receive their gifts. For a gift to be a gift, it must be offered and not taken without permission. To prepare myself for harvesting, I ask myself the following questions:

- Am I in a good frame of mind and heart?
- Have I asked for permission from the local Indigenous community?
- Am I prepared for my harvest?
- Am I harvesting in a good area, free from contaminants?
- Do I know how to spread out my harvest so that I leave enough for non-human life and for the plants to thrive and regenerate?

Asking Permission from the Local Indigenous Community

The practice of giving a territorial acknowledgment, or naming the Indigenous lands you are on, has become a much more common and expected protocol when holding events or activities on Indigenous lands. Though this practice is important, it does not stand alone. It requires associated action to hold true meaning. One way to do this is to consider what activities one can do to support local Indigenous communities. One action we can all take is to learn whose traditional territory we live on. If we are wanting to harvest, we can ask permission and become familiar with culturally important areas we shouldn't harvest in. We can also ask if there is a way to give back. Is there a youth group that might want to come out harvesting? Is there an elders group that could benefit from you sharing your harvest? Perhaps you should not harvest a certain plant, and instead look at growing it yourself or sourcing it from a native plant nursery. I ask permission when I am outside my home territory, especially if I am harvesting a culturally important plant food or medicine. This ensures that I am considering the people from that land before my own harvesting desires.

Preparing for a Harvest

Follow the steps below before setting out to harvest:

1. Familiarize yourself with how to identify the plant, when it is ready for harvest, and what a sustainable harvest looks like. Ask, "How do I give back to this plant and to the land where it grows?"

2. Plan for how to process the plant once you have harvested it. A strong teaching is not to take too much and to be sure to use all that you harvest.

3. Do you have the proper equipment to harvest this plant? Please see the guidelines on the next pages for a list of materials you may want to collect.

Plant Harvesting and Cultivating Materials

Before you head out into the garden or forest, consider what you may need from the following lists:

PLANT IDENTIFICATION

Must-Haves:

- Selection of plant field guides that have clear photographs, taxonomic identification keys, and other important information on habitat and timing of planting/cultivating/harvesting.

Good-to-Haves:

- Plant press for making herbarium pressings to aid in identification and to record areas where particular plants are found growing.

- Magnifying lens or loupe for closer inspection of small plant parts for identification purposes.

- Soft measuring tape if you would like to verify identification measurements in field guides.

PLANT HARVESTING EQUIPMENT

Must-Haves:

- Good harvesting basket or breathable bag. Baskets are one of my obsessions for good reason! They allow for airflow, come in many different shapes and sizes, and are structured enough to create some protection for delicate plant materials. They are also multipurpose, as they can carry your field guide and snacks.

- Drying rack with good airflow and a suitable surface for securely drying plants. You can make your own from window screens or purchase herb-drying racks from garden stores.

Good-to-Haves:

- Gloves for harvesting plants with thorns, stinging hairs, or phototoxic compounds (naturally occurring chemicals in plants that react with sunlight to cause a skin reaction).

- Clippers for cutting through larger woody stems or plants that have stinging hairs, such as stinging nettle.

- Sturdy harvesting knife that you can store safely and that you don't mind getting dirty.

- Digging stick if you have access to one; these traditional tools are very helpful for digging precisely and carefully without disturbing other plant roots.

SAFETY EQUIPMENT

Must-Haves:

- First aid kit stocked for remote settings.

- Bear spray if in areas where bears live.

- Means of communication other than cell phone if out of range (satellite phone, radio).

- Trip plan that can be left with someone at home so they know where you are going and when you plan to return; this is especially important if you are going further afield to harvest.

- Extra layers and rain gear for changing weather.

- Water and food.

PLANT CULTIVATION MATERIALS

Must-Haves:

- Seeds or plant starters from your local native plant nursery, or seeds you have collected.

- Pots, raised beds, or garden beds. Many native plants thrive in containers and pots; growing your own plants helps take harvesting pressure off wild plant populations and also creates habitat and food in your garden for wildlife such as birds and insects. This also may allow you to save seeds or share starts with local Indigenous communities.

Good-to-Haves:

- Gardening gloves.

- Seed markers to record where you are planting seeds.

- Gardening book or resources to help you prepare your soils and plant native plants in ideal conditions.

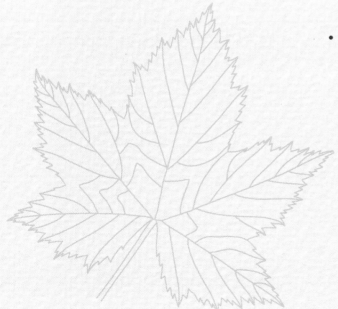

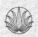 ## Knowing Your Harvest Sites

Finding places to harvest plants can take some time and exploration. Once you have permission and know what plant you are intending to harvest, you can set out to find those special places on the land to build relationships with plants and eventually harvest them. This may be a site in your own garden, that of a friend or family member, or a community garden. Considering alternatives to wild harvesting is a way of sustainable harvesting. When exploring harvest sites, you can look for signs that the area is far away from potential sources of contamination such as major roads, power lines, industrial sites, and dog parks. If you are planning to dry your plants, it is important to select your harvest areas carefully. You don't want to wash leaves, flowers, bark, or any plant part you are going to be drying, as adding extra water to delicate petals, leaves, or shoots can increase the chances of mold and rancidity when storing and utilizing the botanicals later. Know the cultural significance of areas in your region and be respectful. Take care not to harvest in traditional harvesting grounds, and not to harvest plant species that are endangered, rare, or spiritually significant, as you need to have training and cultural context to safely and respectfully utilize such botanicals.

Spreading Out Your Harvest and Leaving Enough Behind

The ways you spread out your harvest will depend on if you are harvesting shoots, leaves, flowers, roots, or bark. Remember, a key sustainable harvesting practice is to not take too much; don't take the first plant you encounter or the last of a particular plant. Overharvesting is a real concern and has a detrimental impact on wild plant populations. Plants such as stinging nettle, wild leeks, and ostrich fern fiddleheads have all been put under great pressure due to their popularity with wild food foragers, chefs, and related businesses. Medicinal and spiritual plants such as white sage, palo santo, and the yew tree have faced severe (and in some cases ongoing) pressures due to popularization and commercialization. When botanicals become popularized without any cultural context of lived experience, it is frighteningly easy for humans to quickly overburden or exploit culturally important plants to the brink of extinction, and certainly to inhibit the access of cultural groups who rely on the plant for ancestral health and wellness practices.

Understanding the life cycle of a plant can help inform you how to spread out your harvest sustainably. Again, remember not to take the first plant you happen upon, don't take more than you need or can use, certainly don't take more than half a stand of a plant, and be sure to make an offering and give back to the plant or the land in any way you can. For example, when I harvest wild rose petals, I'm careful to leave two to three petals on each rose flower so that pollinators can still land upon it. With plants that reroot themselves, such as willow and devil's club, cuttings can be planted in the place of the plant you harvested. Spreading root segments from plants such as camas and rice root while you harvest will enhance their reproduction, and saving or spreading seeds will ensure culturally important plants come back year after year.

 ## While I Harvest

The following teachings in relation to harvesting have been shared with me by elders and family members over the years. I offer them here as a starting place for you to consider your own teachings or traditions:

1 Introduce myself to the plant.

2 Share my intention to harvest the plant in a mindful and respectful way.

3 Ask permission to harvest and listen to the response.

4 Make an offering to the plant.

5 Enact reciprocity toward the plant; this could be to replant part of the plant, spread its seeds, grow the plant in my garden, and plant more plants in its place.

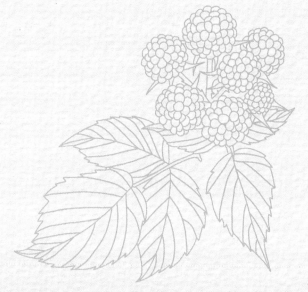

Introducing Myself and Sharing My Intention

I've been taught to introduce myself in my Indigenous language so that the ancestors can understand me. This is an act that is personal to me and that I carry out even when I'm outside of my home territory, as it feels meaningful to ground my mindful presence in my cultural language. As a child, I witnessed my elders and relatives in conversation with non-human life—my great-uncle speaking to the plants in his garden, my father speaking to the deer he just harvested, my great-aunt speaking to the medicines she prepared—so it doesn't feel unfamiliar to now be practicing speaking with plants and teaching my children to do so. Taking the time and care to introduce yourself to a plant is a way of showing respect, and it also acknowledges your intentions. Making the time to do this can cue a deeper awareness of the surrounding area and give you time to observe if the plant looks healthy and plentiful. Are there signs of other recent harvests? Are you near or in a culturally significant site?

During my introduction, I also share my intentions: to be respectful, to listen, to be grateful, and to utilize all that I harvest to create food, medicine, or material that carries with it love and honor for the plant itself.

Making an Offering and Enacting Reciprocity

Making an offering is a personal act that can and should be grounded in your own cultural or personal practices and beliefs. This is an act that embodies reciprocity and can be informed by your own relationship with the plant you are harvesting. When I harvest, I introduce myself, make an offering of tobacco, and share my intention with the plant. I don't take too much, and I give back by replanting part of the plant or growing it in my garden as a way of reducing the harvesting pressure on wild plant populations. This is an opportunity to invite ceremony and ritual into building your relationships with plants. I don't mean you should appropriate or borrow ceremony; rather, connect to your own traditions or cultural practices or explore practical ways to contribute to sustainably harvesting and rebuilding wild plant populations. If you don't know your traditions or cultural practices, this may be an opportunity to seek out a family or community member and ask them. Many unexpected things can come when we take these kinds of risks and opportunities.

Asking Permission and Listening to the Answer: Teachings from Ch'átyaý for a Mindful Harvest

I have had experiences in my life linked to learning from ch'átyaý (devil's club) as a teacher. The first was a few years ago when I was teaching an ethnobotany course on Haida Gwaii at the Kay Llnagaay heritage center in Skidegate as a visitor on Haida territory. I was co-instructing the course with a Haida teacher, which was important to me as an Indigenous instructor from another territory. The day before the course started, I went for a walk on a trail close to Skidegate. Excited and wanting to bring some plants into the classroom with me on the first day, I set out to respectfully harvest from a handful of culturally important plants. I had salmonberry, cedar, lichen, and ch'átyaý in mind. I had brought my tobacco to make an offering to the plants as I introduced myself to them, told them where I am from, and what my intention was in harvesting from them. I located the first three plants fairly quickly and felt confident harvesting a small amount as the stands were thriving in and around the forest area I was hiking in. I kept coming across wet depressions in the forest where ch'átyaý should have been growing, yet there wasn't a plant in sight. As I made my way further up the trail, I puzzled at the lack of ch'átyaý growing in the area. Then a feeling came over me as if someone gently tapped my elbow, and it was clear: the message I was hearing was I was not invited to harvest this plant here.

When I received this message, I thanked the forest and the carrier of the message and turned to hike back down to the trail to bring the other plants home and put them in water for the class the following day. I had only taken a few steps when I saw a large ch'átyaý plant out of the corner of my eye, growing just in the place I would have expected it to grow. I looked beyond and saw a handful of other plants scattered throughout the forest understory. It felt undeniable in that moment that, knowing my intention to harvest it, the plant had hidden itself from me. Once I had received the message that the answer was no, it revealed itself.

Now, my logical brain started explaining the coincidence; it told me that sometimes the trail looks different on the way down, and perhaps I was so focused on certain areas that I missed the places that the scarce single plants were growing. But I knew this wasn't the case. I felt it. When I asked my Haida co-instructor about the state of ch'átyaý on the islands, she told me it was declining rapidly due to over-browsing from introduced deer, and that people were feeling sadness at seeing this important medicine decline. She reaffirmed that it was a good thing I didn't harvest any. I learned two lessons there. As a visitor in an area, it is so important to not only ask permission from the plants, but also from the Indigenous stewards of the land. I knew this! And I felt foolish having not taken that step, so that was one reminder. But I also learned what it feels like to ask permission to harvest and to be told NO.

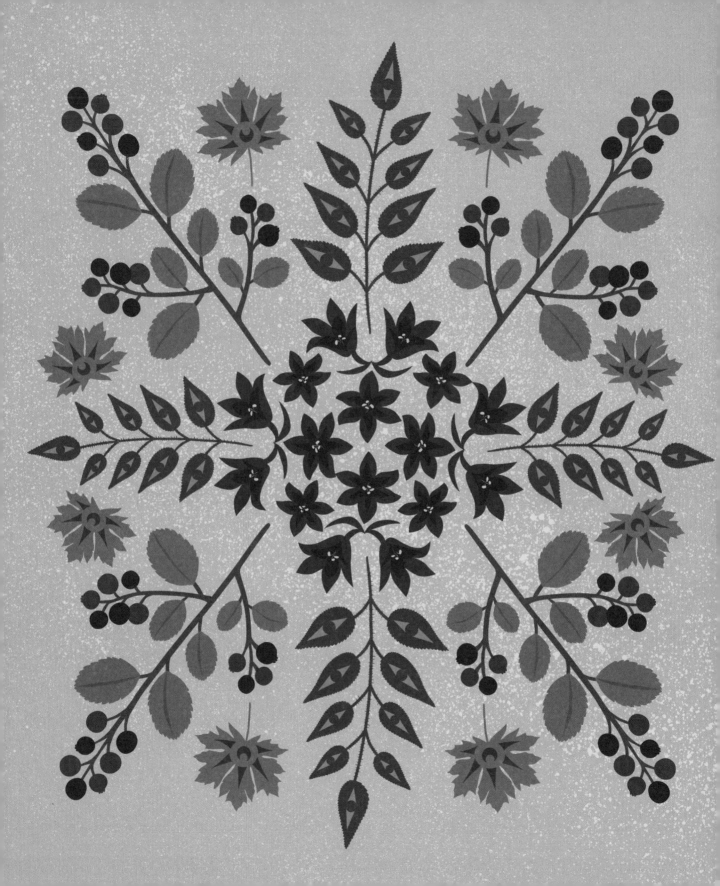

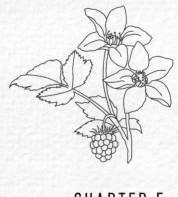

CHAPTER 5

Botanical or Land-Based Mindfulness Practices

In this section, I will introduce steps and considerations for developing your very own botanical or land-based mindfulness practices. I have found these hugely supportive and helpful in my life, and it is my hope and intention to share a framework that you as a reader can meaningfully integrate into your life.

I will outline the steps and framework here so that you can familiarize yourself with them and start to develop your own practices. I would first like to share a bit about my experiences with learning about mindfulness and meditation, and the role that both practices play in my life. A starting point is to begin to pay attention to the cues and indicators in your natural environment. The first section will encourage ways to do this. Then, I invite you to adapt the ideas here to fit the region where you live and the places that are significant to you.

Noticing Nature

It wasn't that long ago that our time was guided by the rhythms and cycles of the natural world. I love thinking about the time when my ancestors would have been so in touch with their natural environment that the seasons and life cycles of plants and other non-human life would have guided their entire concept of time. One of the ways I've built my connection to the natural world is to notice the botanical indications of seasonality in my surroundings.

More and more, I mark the changing of the seasons by noticing subtle botanical cues. I stand at my window in early June and notice the feathery wisps of kw'enikwáy (cottonwood) seeds drifting in the air, catching sunlight and glinting as they are carried on the warm breeze. Traveling on the wind, as they have evolved to do, to the places that will become their homes.

Plants have evolved survival strategies and interrelationships that span everything from how to attract pollinators, gather required nutrients, capture water and light, and in some cases to retain water during drought or extreme temperatures. Plants are incredible teachers. They have so much to teach us if we are willing to listen, observe, and build our own relationships with them. It is the interconnectedness of plants and fungi with their natural surroundings that I invite you to remember throughout the rest of this section. As we look at developing our land-based mindfulness practices, we can consider the interconnections in nature and know that when we are in respectful relationship with the land and with plants, we too are connected.

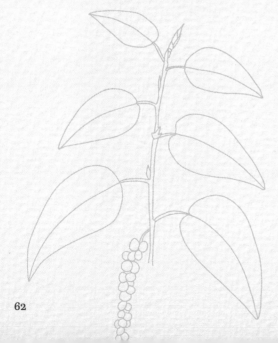

Mindfulness and Meditation

I want to preface this section by stating that often practices of mindfulness and meditation are not necessarily approached in a way that is informed by and sensitive to trauma. As an Indigenous woman, I have found mindfulness and meditation extremely helpful in my life, including in facing the impacts of my experiences with racism and intergenerational trauma. However, it can be very difficult and may stir up strong emotions or triggers when we sit with ourselves in mindful ways. In this section, I share my story of integrating these practices into my life through a lens of plant relationships. I hope that what I share resonates for you, the reader. If you are interested in learning more about mindfulness and meditation but are concerned about facing difficult internal issues, I encourage you to find practitioners who gently integrate mindfulness and meditation in a way that is appropriate for those affected by trauma.

I feel things deeply in life—the good, the bad, and the in-between. I believe that this feeling *into* life experiences and situations helps me to access a presence in the moment, and glimpses of an intuitive understanding of what it means for me, Leigh Joseph, to be alive at this moment in time. That is not to say that it helps me decode the great unknown that we all face as humans, or reduce the uncertainty of the future. Instead, it helps me to trust more in the process, trust in the moment, and know that this moment—good or bad or in-between—will not last forever. This acknowledgment of the ever-changing and sometimes fleeting nature of the moments that make up our lives is both beautiful and potentially overwhelming.

As one of my teachers shared with me, mindfulness can be found in the mundane daily rituals: waking up, making coffee, dressing for the day, walking, driving to school or work, or preparing food. These are just some examples that I share to emphasize that mindfulness does not need to come with significant events or experiences, but can be accessed in the moments that make up our days, our lives, our stories. Mindfulness is a practice of bringing awareness and presence of mind and thought to a moment: taking a single breath in through your nose and exhaling that breath out of your mouth. This act, when mindful attention is brought to it, has the power to deescalate racing thoughts and ease fight-or-flight responses in the body. Mindful breath can expand mental and emotional spaciousness, and this is beneficial if even just for a moment. After all, our lives are made up of a collection of moments that are unique to us as individuals.

Land-Based Mindfulness

Land-based mindfulness practices are ones that can be put into action outdoors, and can be enhanced through the development of, and in combination with, land-based visualizations.

Later in this chapter, I share a land-based visualization related to harvesting stinging nettle, as well as steps for a land-based mindfulness practice connected to the visualization. The visualization is meant to transport you in your mind to a place on the land anytime it is supportive for you to do so. Land-based mindfulness practices can be done outdoors and build off the visualizations through actually connecting with the land physically. The interplay between land-based visualizations and land-based mindfulness practices can help support mental, emotional, spiritual, and physical health, and can be tailored to you and your relationships with the land and with place.

The following are general steps to develop land-based mindfulness practices. Remember, mindfulness can come in the small moments and the daily acts that we all experience. By bringing mindful awareness to connecting to nature and outdoor spaces, one can cultivate practices that can support you year-round, either indoors or out.

1 Visit a place outdoors that is special or significant to you.

2 Take off your shoes and feel your feet on the ground.

3 Run your hands over the trees or plants around you.

4 Smell the plants, the leaves, the flowers, the bark.

5 Breathe the air.

6 Notice how the ground and air *feel*.

7 Is it cold outside? Warm, hot?

8 Is there a breeze?

9 What does the sun, rain, or shade feel like on your skin?

10 What can you hear? Birds, water, people?

Following these steps can help to ground you in a place and moment in time. Feeling connected to the larger natural world is a way we can support ourselves and also consider how we can give back in reciprocity and respect to the natural world.

Visualization

Visualization can complement mindfulness and meditation practices by offering a touchstone to help ground you in moments of mindful awareness. Examples include visualizing breath as color or visualizing a special place that brings you comfort. I have found that having a place out on the land that I can envision easily and in detail has helped me to develop visualizations that support my mindfulness and meditation practices.

For me, these visualizations are connected to both being on the land and to being in relationship with plants. I have practiced visiting a special or significant place on the land in my mind's eye; the more detailed the visualization is, the easier it is to revisit this place mentally, and the more grounding the exercise. Sensory aspects such as scents, temperature, and sounds can bring details that can help you immerse yourself in that place.

Steps for Developing Your Own Land-Based Visualization

1 Make a list of places on the land that are or have been important in your life. This could be a childhood garden or camping spot or a favorite trail or a sacred site. Think of the places that come to mind and settle on one that feels grounding, safe, and supportive.

2 Consider if there are people important to you who are connected to this place. How does it feel to be in their presence?

3 Make a list of the details of the place. In what season do you visit this place? What can you hear nearby?

4 Start by writing out your visualization of this place. You can open your written visualization with "I walk into the forest . . ." or "I sit on the ground and look up at the trees . . ." Find a way to enter this place in your mind. Writing out your visualization will help you to clearly outline the place so in the future you can access it in your mind's eye more easily.

5 Picture the plants that are growing there and spend time envisioning the details of the plants. Do the leaves have a scent? Are the flowers a certain color? If that plant is edible, what does it taste like?

Following these prompts can help you to develop your visualization, which in turn can support your overall mindfulness and meditation practices.

Land-Based Mindfulness Practice for Ḵáⱡḵay (Wild Rose) Harvest

I arrive at my favorite ḵáⱡḵay harvesting spot and get out my basket. I walk into the estuary. I put my tobacco offering down at the base of the first ḵáⱡḵay plant I find. Then I keep walking for a while to see how many ḵáⱡḵay plants are in the area so I can be sure there are enough plants growing here to support my harvest. I place my basket somewhere nearby that is easy to find. (I have misplaced harvesting items before, and it can take a long time to find them again.) Then I start the following steps.

1   I ground myself on the land. I feel the support of the earth beneath me, knowing I am held, I am connected, I am part of the earth.

2   I take three slow breaths in through my nose and out through my mouth to ground myself.

3   I become still, perhaps sitting down comfortably and leaning against a tree for support. I slow my breathing; I feel the air come in through my nose and out through my mouth. I repeat this to the count of ten.

4   I feel into the areas of my body that are in contact with the earth, and I feel my back leaning against the tree. I imagine my energy extending down into the earth, connecting with the roots, rhizomes, and mycorrhiza. I imagine energy moving out from the crown of my head and connecting with the warm spring air, allowing itself to be carried on the gentle breeze. I see myself as connected to nature.

5   I start to notice the sounds I can hear: the birds around me, the scent of ḵáⱡḵay petals in the sun, the rustling of branches and leaves as the breeze moves through them. I hear my children playing nearby, laughing, chattering, and gently speaking with the plants.

6   Next, I notice the scents in the air: the smell of the soil, the warm scent of summer, and the plants that are growing in and around the area—ḵálḵay, yarrow, sweet gale.

7   I turn inward and notice how I feel in my body. I feel into my jaw, relaxing it. Then I relax my face, my head and neck, down to my shoulders, my chest, into my belly, my hips and legs, my ankles and feet, down my arms, and into my hands. I notice what I feel with each breath in and out as I survey my body.

8   From this place, I bring my attention back to my breath. In and out. I start to focus only on this breath. In and out. Connected outside, on the land. Aware of being safe, held, present.

9   I stay this way for as long as feels good, or I may have a timer to bring gentle structure to my land-based mindfulness practice.

10 Once I close my practice, I will come back into the current moment and relish the foundation of quiet, mindful presence that I cultivated. I will carry this with me into the day and into my harvest.

This practice may last a few minutes or much longer if you have the space to extend your time. When thoughts arise you can notice them and then refocus on your breath. Be gentle with yourself.

Land-Based Visualization for Ts'exts'íx (Stinging Nettle)

I will now share one of my land-based botanical mindfulness visualizations here in connection with my favorite nettle-harvesting area to illustrate how land-based visualizations and mindfulness practices can connect. When you are not able to be out on the land, you can still access these moments, and the benefits of your land-based and place-based relationships, in your mind's eye.

I close my eyes and am transported to a stretch of forest about 8 miles (5 km) north from my house. This is the place I come to harvest stinging nettle with my family in the spring. The sun is shining as we unpack our baskets, clippers, and gloves from the car. I can see the dappled sunlight coming through the new leaves of the cottonwood and red alder trees. I can smell the damp earth that is still warming up from the cool overnight temperatures. There is still some dew on the plants. I can see the earth through the emerging blanket of vibrant green. Salmonberry and thimbleberry shoots crop up. Yellow stream violets and miner's lettuce stand in juicy, lush, cushion-like stands. And then there is the deep green of the ts'exts'íx, the chlorophyll-rich tender new shoots coming into focus as I train my eyes to discern them among all the green. I close my eyes. I can feel the slight chill in the air and the warmth of the spring sun all at once. I hear my children laughing not too far off. The more distant sound of the Squamish River is almost indistinguishable from the gentle sound of the breeze through the alder leaves. I feel grounded in this place. I feel at ease, joyful, safe. I introduce myself to the plant relation that I am harvesting today, saying:

Ts'exts'íx, Ha7lh skwáyel! Styawat kwi nkwsh min. Skwxwú7mesh Úxwumixw. An wanxwstn skwálwen i7xw ten s7ekw' 7tel.

(ha-th sk-why-al! sty-ah-wat kw-i en kw-sh-aw-main. sk-xw-o-mesh oh-xw-oh may-xw. an wan-ow-xws en skw-al-wen eh-xw ten se-kw-eh-tal.)

Good day, my ancestral name is Styawat, I come from the Squamish Nation. I'm happy to be here, my heart is full. All my relations.

I ask permission to harvest, and I leave an offering to the plant. The answer is yes. I gently clip the tender green shoots and place them in my harvesting basket, spreading out and only taking small numbers from each stand. My ankle brushes against the stinging hairs, and I jump at the bite of this plant. It reminds me of the medicine and the care that needs to be taken when harvesting this plant in a respectful way. My children are there, rolling around like bear cubs, laughing, feeling free and safe. This is a place that brings me peace and ease, and I visit it in my mind time and time again to find grounding and strength.

 ## Plant Processing and Mindfulness

Your mindful engagement with plants can span beyond the harvest and into the processing of, and eventually creating with, plant ingredients. All plants will require some processing once they are harvested. I have been taught that it is important to do this as soon as possible so as not to risk the plants rotting. Otherwise, this would be considered a waste and a disrespect to the plant.

When you process a plant, it may be that you are separating the outer bark from the inner bark or the leaves from the stem, or cleaning or removing debris or parts of the plant you don't want to use. In the case of spruce tips, there is a papery brown sheath that I like to remove while I harvest as it is difficult to remove later. This sheath isn't dangerous, but it does change the flavor of an infused spruce tip syrup, for example. With rosehips, you need to remove the hairy seeds inside the fruit before eating them. The processing of plant materials takes time and care and provides another opportunity for mindful engagement. While you process the plant, you can think back to tending and harvesting it. You can build a land-based visualization in connection to the plant. If the plant is aromatic or edible, you can crush some of it between your fingers and inhale the scent. If it is edible, you can place a small amount on your tongue and let the flavor transport you. Then, later, if you are making a recipe with dried botanicals that you have harvested, you can also follow these same steps to reconnect with the feeling of tending and harvesting the plant.

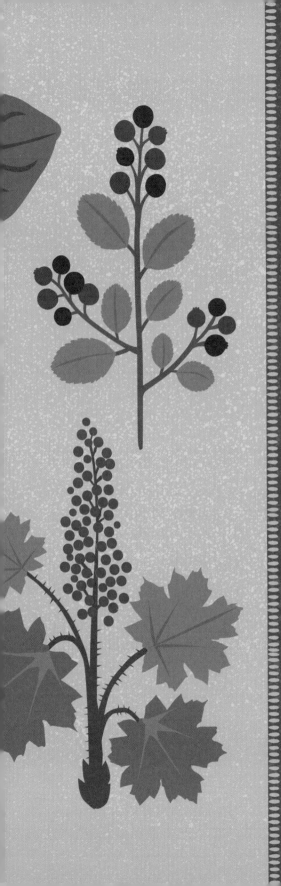

PLANT
*Profiles &
Recipes*

BEING *in* RELATIONSHIP

···◄—◉—►···

Ekw'í7tel—*to be related*

I mention relationship between people and plants throughout this book, as I see relationship as central to learning about, and eventually utilizing, plants in nutrition, wellness, and beauty practices. To me, being in relationship with plants means identifying how to uphold my side of the partnership in respectful and reciprocal ways. This may be in how I can give back to the plant through replanting seeds or root segments. Perhaps I grow the plant in my garden and save some to plant in the land. I have been taught that when we work with plants to create food, medicine, or material, it is important to be in a good frame of mind and heart, as how you are feeling goes into what you are creating.

In this section I will go into more detail about forty-four culturally important plants that grow in Squamish Territory or that have been culturally important to my community. Each plant profile is designed to:

- introduce you to the plant through a personal reflection or experience
- share the Squamish, English, and Latin plant names
- help you identify the plant and learn about its habitat
- include a recipe to make with the plant, either for culinary or beauty purposes

I chose to approach these plant profiles specifically through my lens as a Squamish woman, as opposed to attempting to capture a wide range of different Indigenous knowledge and practices connected to each plant. There is such a richness and diversity across Indigenous Peoples and communities and their relationships and knowledge connected to plants. I encourage any reader to explore further ethnobotanical knowledge connected to plants they are particularly interested in. The ranges of most of the plants included here are vast and will cover many different Indigenous territories as well as ecological zones. Some of the plants have a variety of species that are closely related but vary slightly by region. However, some (wild rose, for example) are utilized in mostly the same ways regardless of the exact species. It is my hope that my stories and the information shared in this book are relevant and helpful to a broader audience, especially other Indigenous individuals and communities who are working to reconnect with cultural knowledge and practices.

Although illustrations have been provided to aid with identification, it is vitally important to read the entire plant profile before attempting to harvest or grow any plant. The text contains details that are crucial for accurate identification. I have also added in warnings for plants that require care in harvesting, processing, or preparation. Please read these warnings thoroughly and remember never to harvest or ingest a plant that you are not one hundred percent comfortable identifying and preparing properly. For further information on harvesting plants in a safe and ethical manner, please refer to the "Cautions, Warnings, and Responsibilities" section on page 13.

Some recipes include optional ingredients or materials you can use to enhance the final dish or product. These options should be considered as suggestions and I encourage you to be creative. Please note that some of the topical recipes include the option to utilize essential oils. Remember to use these oils with care. All essential oils should be used in moderation.

Legend

Indicates this plant should be handled with caution

Indicates a recipe used for topical/beauty purposes only

Indicates a culinary recipe

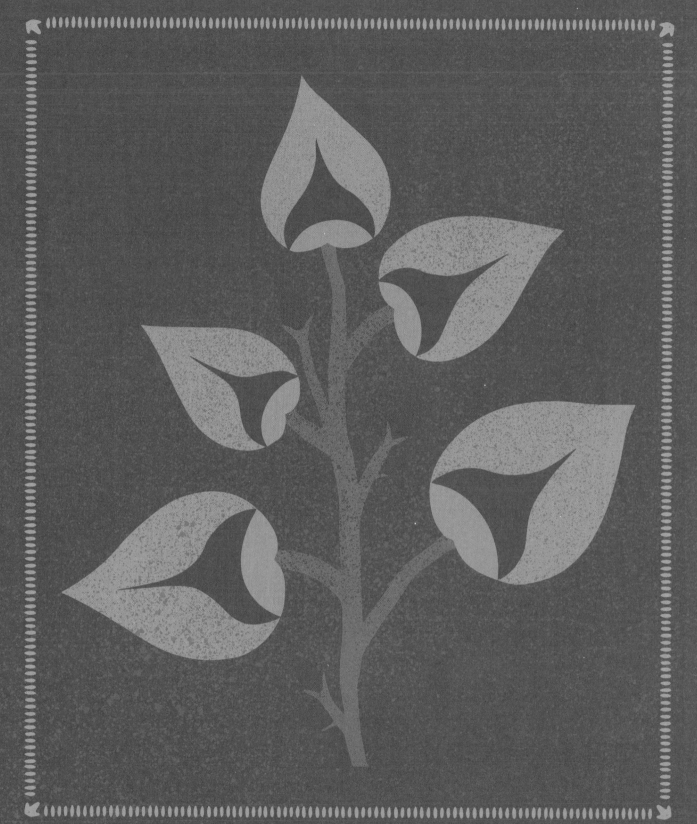

TREES

...◄●►...

Kwéxwmáy

kw-ex-wm-eye

AMABILIS FIR

Abies amabilis

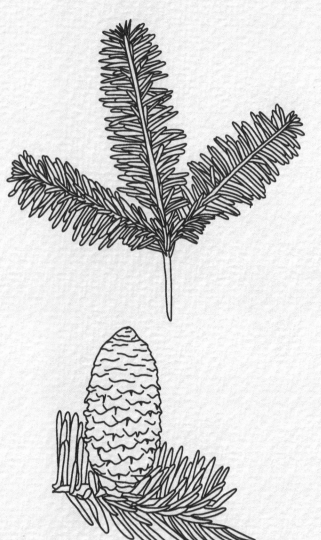

BUILDING RELATIONSHIPS

This is a special tree to me. My paternal grandmother, Rose, used the medicine obtained from this tree to support her health. It is one of the first tree medicines I remember learning about as a child. My dad told me that his mom was taught to squeeze, and deeply inhale directly from, the tree's resin-filled blisters. Each year I travel into the higher elevations in Skwxwú7mesh to harvest this golden treasure. The resin or pitch of this tree has the most incredible scent, and after a full day of harvesting I may leave with ½–1 cup of resin. This harvest is a labor of love and has become a favorite for me and my family.

HABITAT

Kwéxwmáy grows most commonly in cool, moist forest sites with deep, well-drained soils and is very tolerant of shade. Kwéxwmáy is found from southwestern British Columbia (BC), except Haida Gwaii, down to the Cascade Mountains in Washington and Oregon and to Northern California. It's found at higher elevations (above 3,280 feet, or 1,000 m) in southern BC and in lower elevations in the central and northern regions of its range.

BOTANICAL DESCRIPTION

Kwéxwmáy is a tall, straight tree that grows to approximately 180 feet (55 m) in height with a dense cylindrical, round-topped crown. The young bark is whitish gray with resin-filled blisters, and turns scaly with age. The needles are 0.5–1 inch (1.5–2.5 cm) long, and are flat, with blunt, notched tips. They are dark green on top with a silvery underside, and two distinct bands of stomata underneath. Some needles are found on top of the twigs and point forward, which differentiates it from grand fir. Branches are flat and spray-like. Seed cones are 3–6 inches (8–15 cm) long and 1–2 inches (2.5–5 cm) thick and are deep purple, barrel-shaped, and stand straight up on the branch. The pollen cones are small and reddish.

SUSTAINABLE HARVEST AND TIMING

It is part of our responsibility when harvesting tree resin to remember that the resin serves to protect the tree itself. Each time we score the bark of a tree, we are exposing it to potential risk of infection or infestation, so it is important to harvest carefully and sparingly and to rotate harvesting areas year after year. The resin can be harvested in any season.

PLANT GIFTS

The bark has resin-filled blisters that are characteristic of this tree and its relatives. The blisters hold antibacterial and antimicrobial sap that protects the tree. However, this beautifully aromatic resin also has multiple benefits for humans when used topically and internally. When the resin is sustainably harvested with care and infused into a carrier oil or tasted fresh from the bark, it carries medicinal effects that are beneficial to us humans. The resin from conifers like kwéxwmáy helps to support healing and can be used topically on minor cuts and scrapes. The needles have a wonderful citrusy flavor that lends itself well to culinary recipes. For recipes like the one below, pick the new growth of the branches, or the tips, in the spring when they are tender.

Salmon Baked in Kwéxwmáy Tips and Lemon

2 servings

½ cup (63 g) fresh or frozen kwéxwmáy tips or spruce tips (defrosted if frozen)
½ lemon, zested
¼ cup (60 ml) mayonnaise (you can also substitute for equal amounts tahini or pesto as dairy-free options)
1 tablespoon olive oil
¼ teaspoon salt
2 salmon fillets (around 5 ounces, or 140 g each)

1   Preheat the oven to 350°F (175°C).

2   Roughly chop the kwéxwmáy tips and add them to a small bowl.

3   Add the lemon zest, mayonnaise, olive oil, and salt. Taste and adjust seasoning as necessary (e.g., add some fresh lemon juice for more citrus flavor). Mix well.

4   Place the salmon fillets skin sides down on a greased baking tray. Spread the mixture of kwéxwmáy tips and mayonnaise evenly over the two fillets.

5   Bake for 13–15 minutes, depending on how thick the salmon is. The salmon should flake easily, and/or register an internal temperature of 145°F (63°C). Remove and let rest for at least 5 minutes before enjoying.

Ḵ'emeláy

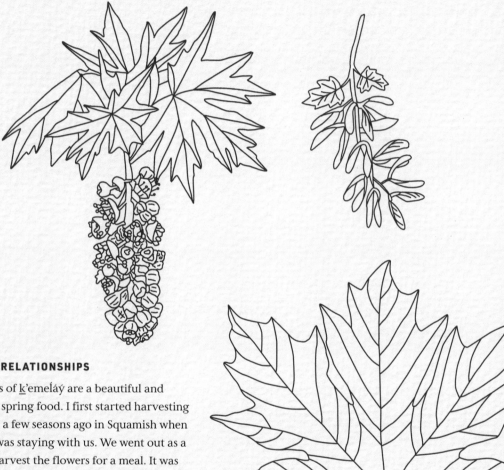

BUILDING RELATIONSHIPS

The flowers of ḵ'emeláy are a beautiful and substantial spring food. I first started harvesting the flowers a few seasons ago in Squamish when my father was staying with us. We went out as a family to harvest the flowers for a meal. It was his job to jump up and pull the branches down so the kids and I could reach the ḵ'emeláy flowers and place them in our baskets. I can still see him jumping up like a basketball player and gently pulling the branches down to his grandchildren's reaching hands. Time spent on the land with loved ones creates special memories.

HABITAT

K̲'emeĺáy grows at low to mid elevations in mesic to moist mixed coniferous and deciduous forests, as well as on open, rocky sites, especially alongside Douglas fir, red alder, and red cedar. It occurs commonly in southwestern BC and south to California, mostly west of the Pacific coast and the Cascade Mountains.

BOTANICAL DESCRIPTION

K̲'emeĺáy is a medium to large sized tree growing up to 115 feet (35 m) tall with a broad, rounded crown. Its bark is smooth and green when young, but turns gray-brown and ridged with age and is often covered with moss and ferns. Leaves are large, five-lobed, and 6–12 inches (15–30 cm) across. Flowers are numerous, greenish-yellow, and hang down in clusters that appear on the branches before the leaves unfurl.

SUSTAINABLE HARVEST AND TIMING

Because you are harvesting the flowers, it is important not to take too many from one tree. However, most of the flowers will be out of reach higher up in the tree; those will be available for pollination and for insects and animals that rely on the blooms. The flowers are harvested in early to mid-April. The sap can be harvested with a tap and bucket, just as with sugar maple sap.

PLANT GIFTS

The k̲'emeĺáy flowers are a lovely early-spring harvest. They are a flavorful and substantial addition to a meal. The Squamish name k̲'emeĺáy translates to "paddle tree"; as a source of hardwood, it was traditionally used to make paddles, as well as other technologies like spindle whorls and tools for processing the inner bark of western red cedar. Many of my relatives use the k̲'emeĺáy wood for smoking salmon as the smoke carries a great flavor.

K̲'emeĺáy Flower Fritters

2–4 servings

½–1 cup (120–240 ml) vegetable oil, or enough to fill your pan with 3–4 inches (7–10 cm) of oil
1 cup (125 g) all-purpose flour
1 teaspoon baking powder
2 eggs, beaten
1 tablespoon cornstarch
About 8 tablespoons (120 ml) ice-cold water
2 cups (40 g) rinsed k̲'emeĺáy flowers
Pinch of herbs and seasoning, or icing sugar if you prefer sweet (optional)
Savory Dipping Sauce (page 181), for serving (optional)

1   In a large skillet, heat the vegetable oil over medium heat.

2   In a medium bowl, mix the flour, baking powder, eggs, and cornstarch together to make a batter. Add the savory seasoning or icing sugar if using. Make sure to mix well enough to remove lumps.

3   Add enough ice-cold water, a tablespoon at a time, until the batter is liquid.

4   Add the rinsed k̲'emeĺáy flowers and stir gently to coat them in batter.

5   Remove the flowers from the batter and place them in the hot pan, making sure to space them out.

6   Fry until golden brown on each side. Serve with the Savory Dipping Sauce or on their own.

K̲w'eník̲w'ay

kw-en-eh-kw-eye

BLACK POPLAR OR COTTONWOOD

Populus trichocarpa (also known as *P. balsamifera* ssp. *trichocarpa*)

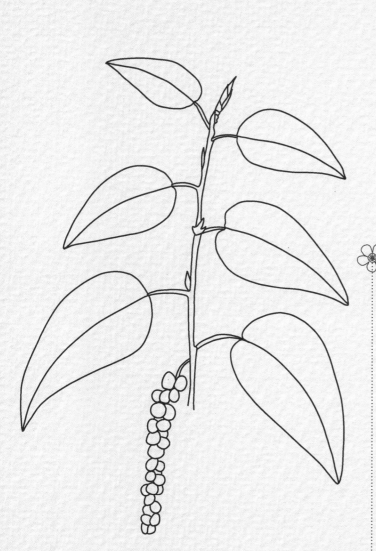

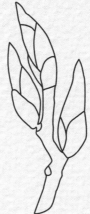

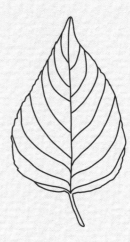

BUILDING RELATIONSHIPS

Each spring when the days start to lengthen and warm up, before most other plants have started to unfurl their leaves and turn the landscape to vibrant green, the k̲w'eník̲w'ay leaf buds start to become plump with golden resin that smells like the sweet warmth of a spring day. When my children were little, this was the first harvest of the spring. My daughter was three years old when she surprised me by identifying the leaf buds of k̲w'eník̲w'ay on the bare branches. If you have ever tried to identify trees before the leaves come out, it can be very difficult. I realized in that moment that my children had been absorbing all their experiences on the land since they were tiny. It made me feel deeply contented knowing that, right then and there, my children and I were rebuilding ancestral knowledge and experiences on the land together.

HABITAT

Ḵw'eníḵw'ay grows in moist to wet riparian habitats including river terraces, floodplains, gravel bars, islands, streambanks, and lakeshores from Alaska along the BC coast, down into the Cascades, and inland to the Rockies.

BOTANICAL DESCRIPTION

Ḵw'eníḵw'ay grows up to 82–131 feet (25–40 m) in height, with big straight trunks and gray bark that is deeply furrowed on mature trees. The large, deciduous leaves are heart-shaped and shiny green. The leaf buds are orange-brown and resinous, fragrant, and sticky to the touch, especially in the spring when temperatures start to warm up. Flowers are numerous in dangling catkins that appear before the leaves, and the seeds are covered in fluffy white hairs.

These trees have separate male and female trees. Two different types of catkins can be found growing on them. The smaller male catkins measure 0.8–1.2 inches (2–3 cm) long and the larger female catkins measure 3–8 inches (8–20 cm) long.

SUSTAINABLE HARVEST AND TIMING

During winter windstorms, ḵw'eníḵw'ay branches often fall to the forest floor. Because the leaf buds set (i.e., appear on the branch) the season before, you can harvest them from these fallen branches. Alternatively, if you harvest leaves from a standing tree, you are effectively pruning the tree. In this case, it is important to spread out your harvest and leave the terminal leaf bud on the branch so the tree can continue to grow. The buds are harvested in the early spring, usually late March/early April, before the leaves unfurl.

PLANT GIFTS

The resin from ḵw'eníḵw'ay is a highly valued medicine that has been utilized around the world for thousands of years where species of cottonwood grow. The leaf buds have anti-inflammatory, antiseptic, and analgesic properties. You can prepare infused oil, ointment, and tea from the leaf buds. The infused oil and ointment can be used topically to reduce pain and inflammation from cuts, scrapes, burns, and other wounds. I learned from a Squamish knowledge holder, Swanámiya-t Diana Billy, that you can apply the infused oil to your chest as a rub to help with congestion.

Sun-Infused Ḵw'eníḵw'ay Oil

2 quarts (2 L)

2 cups (250 g) fresh ḵw'eníḵw'ay buds
2 quarts (2 L) organic carrier oil of your choosing (sweet almond oil, olive oil, and sunflower seed oil are all nice options)

1   Let the fresh ḵw'eníḵw'ay buds sit in a basket overnight to allow any moisture to dissipate.

2   Place the leaf buds into a large jar and cover them with the carrier oil (see page 42 for a list of more carrier oils).

3   Cover the jar with cheesecloth and leave it to sit on a windowsill away from moisture. Allow the ḵw'eníḵw'ay buds to infuse slowly into the oil. You can leave this for 2 weeks for a nice infusion (I've even infused it for 6 months); the leaf buds are so antibacterial they will help preserve the carrier oil as long as there is no moisture introduced. By doing a slow sun infusion, you will not lose the gorgeous scent.

T'ú7xwaý

t-oh-xw-eye

GRAND FIR

Abies grandis

BUILDING RELATIONSHIPS

When I walk through the forests in and around Squamish, the t'ú7xwaý trees stand out immediately because of their distinct dark-green needles. The citrusy scent of fresh, crushed t'ú7xwaý needles fills me with a feeling of being simultaneously energized and calm. Each time I come across a t'ú7xwaý tree, I harvest and dry some needles as they are not widespread in this region. The dried needles make an incredible addition to many recipes sweet and savory. T'ú7xwaý is also useful to many animals for cover and nesting sites. Birds, chipmunks, and squirrels eat the seeds.

HABITAT

T'ú7xwaý grows in dry to moist coniferous and mixed forests, from river flats to mountain slopes, especially in warmer, drier parts of the coast. T'ú7xwaý often accompanies ch'shaý (Douglas fir) at low to mid elevations from southern BC along the coast to Northern California. In Washington and northern Oregon, it spreads east to the Cascade Mountains, and is also found in the Rocky Mountains of Idaho and Montana.

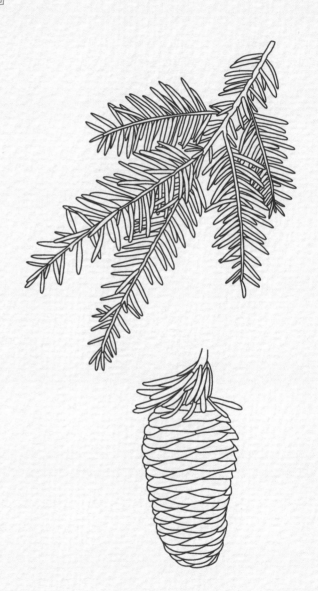

BOTANICAL DESCRIPTION

T'ú7xwaý grows up to 130–260 feet (40–80 m) tall. The needles spread horizontally in two distinct rows and are 1.2–2 inches (3–5 cm) long, deep green in color, shiny, and flat, with rounded, notched tips and two white lines of stomata on the underside. The greenish, cylindric- to barrel-shaped seed cones are 2–4 inches (5–10 cm) long and sit on top of the branch. The pollen cones are small and yellowish. The bark is greyish-brown, often with white mottling, smooth and with resin blisters in younger trees, that becomes ridged and scaly with age.

SUSTAINABLE HARVEST AND TIMING

The resin of t'ú7xwaý can be carefully harvested year-round from younger trees that still have resin blisters on the bark. Care should be taken not to cut into the tree bark beyond piercing the blister to collect the resin in a jar. The boughs can be harvested year-round. You should spread out the harvest across multiple trees so as not to prune too much from one tree.

PLANT GIFTS

The resin of t'ú7xwaý is antibacterial and anti-inflammatory. It can be utilized internally to soothe an upset stomach or applied topically to promote healing for minor skin irritations, cuts, or scrapes. The flavor of the spring tips (the new growth at the ends of the branches) and the mature needles is beautiful and lends itself well to culinary recipes.

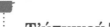

T'ú7xwaý Tip–Crusted Halibut

2 servings

½ cup (72 g) almonds
6–8 t'ú7xwaý tips, chopped, reserving some
    for garnish
2 tablespoons lemon zest
2 tablespoons all-purpose flour
3 tablespoons olive oil
2 halibut fillets (around 5 ounces, or 140 g each)

1   Preheat the oven to 400°F (200°C).

2   Grind up the almonds fine, or a bit chunky if you prefer, in a blender.

3   Toast the ground almonds in a frying pan over medium heat for 3–5 minutes. Keep close by and check often to avoid burning the almonds.

4   Once roasted, place the almonds in a bowl and add in the chopped t'ú7xwaý tips, lemon zest, and flour. Stir together to combine.

5   Place the olive oil on a plate and roll your fish in it to fully coat the fish with oil.

6   Roll the oiled fish in the crust ingredients until coated.

7   Place the crusted fish into a shallow baking dish.

8   Sprinkle the remaining crust ingredients over the fish and bake for 15–20 minutes uncovered. The fish should flake easily, and/or register an internal temperature of 145°F (63°C).

9   Serve, garnished with fresh t'ú7xwaý tips.

<u>K</u>we7úpaý

kw-oh-pa-eye
PACIFIC CRAB APPLE
Malus fusca

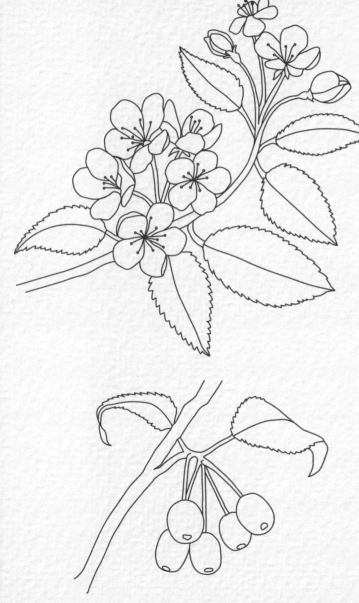

 BUILDING RELATIONSHIPS

<u>K</u>we7úpaý is an important food to the Squamish People and the bark is an important ingredient in an eye wash medicine. The trees have been cultivated in temperate forest gardens in the Pacific Northwest by Indigenous Peoples for thousands of years. The branches of the trees were pruned to allow for ease of harvesting, and the fruit stored in airtight bentwood boxes full of water for use throughout the winter. <u>K</u>we7úpaý fruit was traded and gifted through ceremony, a practice that I have witnessed at recent events and feasts I have attended. Each year in Squamish, my children and I look for these tart fruits along some of our favorite trails and laugh at the sour faces we make when we taste them.

!

WARNING: *<u>K</u>we7úpaý bark contains cyanide-producing compounds and should only be used by trained knowledge holders.*

HABITAT

Kwe7úpaý grows in moist to wet woods, swamps, and edges of standing or flowing water. It often occurs along shorelines and in upper estuaries, at low to mid elevations from Alaska all the way south to California.

BOTANICAL DESCRIPTION

Kwe7úpaý is a multi-stemmed shrub or small tree that ranges from 7–39 feet (2–12 m) in height. The branches have thornlike spur shoots. In spring, blossoms are white to pink in color, and are attractive and fragrant. In fall, the narrowly egg-shaped, toothed leaves turn purplish red or yellow orange, as do the small crab apples.

SUSTAINABLE HARVEST AND TIMING

As with any wild-growing fruit, it is important to leave some for other non-human life that rely on it. Bears eat crab apples, as will some birds. The fruit ripens from late August through September and October.

PLANT GIFTS

The fruit of kwe7úpaý was one of the most important harvests of the later summer and early fall in many Indigenous communities. It was traded and gifted among Indigenous Peoples as, culturally, it was and is so highly regarded. The fruit offers a source of fiber, along with sweetness that only increases when stored (traditionally, submerged in water). The bark of kwe7úpaý trees has been used as an infusion for stomach upset and to soothe various eye ailments.

Low Sugar Kwe7úpaý Honey Jelly

½ cup (170 g)

1 cup (128 g) fresh kwe7úpaý, rinsed and diced
6 cups (1.4 L) water
2 tablespoons honey
2 tablespoons orange juice (or lemon)
1 teaspoon xanthan gum or potato starch

1   Place the kwe7úpaý and water into a medium saucepan, bring to a quick boil, then simmer, covered with the lid, for 1 hour, keeping an eye on the water levels in order not to burn the kwe7úpaý.

2   Take the saucepan off the heat. Mash the kwe7úpaý, along with any remaining liquid, using a potato masher. Then, strain the liquid into a small bowl using a fine sieve, nut bag, or cheesecloth to avoid having any of the seeds as part of your jelly.

3   Place the liquid into a blender and add in the honey, orange juice, and xanthum gum. Blend on low for 10 seconds.

4   Place the jelly in clean, hot canning jars. Wipe the tops of the jars to remove any spillage and cover with the lids.

5   Seal the lids on the jars in a hot-water bath for 10 minutes.

This jelly goes great on wild meats, fish, or over a piece of whole grain bread. Store it for up to 2 months in an airtight glass jar in the cupboard or fridge. If any lids do not seal (see step 5), refrigerate and use within 3 weeks.

Ts'icháýaý

ts-ates-ich-eh-eye

SPRUCE

Picea spp., including
Picea sitchensis and
Picea mariana

 BUILDING RELATIONSHIPS

Ts'icháýaý is an incredibly healing and nourishing tree. It doesn't commonly grow in Squamish, so when I happen upon a tree either during the early spring (spruce tip season) or if I find a crystal of resin on the outer bark, it is a treat. My Squamish ancestors utilized this resin as a healthy gum to chew and utilized the boughs in certain ceremonies. As with any tree identification, it is so helpful to go out repeatedly, bring your field guides or tree identification resources, and take the time to look closely at the needles. Look at how they grow (bundled together or singularly). Crush one and smell the scent. Look at the texture of the bark. Do this for young and older trees.

 HABITAT

The **black spruce** is a northern species that is the dominant tree species in boreal forests across all provinces and territories in Canada, extending north into Alaska and south into Minnesota and Pennsylvania. **White spruce** can be found growing in wet to dry slopes, river terraces, bogs, and fens in the subalpine zone, and grows in central and northern BC, north to Alaska and Yukon, and south into Wyoming and Montana. **Sitka spruce** is found in coastal forests in BC, up into Southeast Alaska, and down to Northern California.

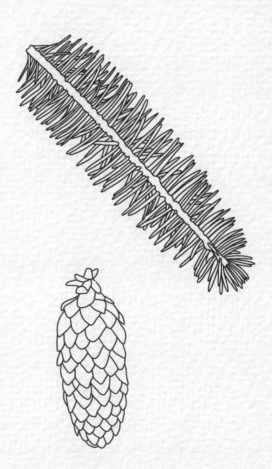

BOTANICAL DESCRIPTION

Ts'icháyaý is an evergreen conifer that ranges in height from 65–295 feet (20–90 m) with conical or spire-like crowns and thin scaly bark. The sharp-tipped needles are 0.4–1.2 inches (1–3 cm) long and grow in a spiral around all sides of the branch. All spruces have seed cones with thin, stiff-papery or somewhat woody but flexible scales that are on the trees from May to July.

SUSTAINABLE HARVEST AND TIMING

When harvesting ts'icháyaý tips, it is important to leave the terminal spruce tip—the tip of the very end of the branch—as this is where the tree's branches will grow out each year in the mid-spring. Spread out the harvest across many different trees so as not to over-prune, and leave tips for other animals that rely on them for food.

When harvesting dried pitch or resin from the outside of the bark, be sure not to take too much from one tree. Pitch can be harvested year-round.

NOTE: *All the equipment you use to harvest and process spruce pitch will be covered in it forever!*

PLANT GIFTS

Ts'icháyaý is full of compounds that smell wonderful and have topical benefits. Elders have shared with me that the pitch heals wounds from the inside out, meaning the antibiotic and antimicrobial properties of the pitch promote healing. I have witnessed this firsthand with the application of spruce pitch to a range of skin irritations, cuts, and scrapes. In the early spring, spruce trees set a bounty of tender new branch tips, the new growth for the year. Spruce tips are a delicious ingredient for many culinary recipes, are rich in vitamin C, and have a delicate citrusy flavor.

Candied Ts'icháyaý Tips

2 cups (250 g) candied tips and 1 quart (1 L) infused syrup

2 cups (250 g) freshly picked ts'icháyaý tips, with the papery brown sheath removed (it is not harmful but will change the flavor)
1 quart (1 L) maple or birch syrup

1 Pour water in the bottom pot of a double boiler, being careful not to have the water touching the bottom of the top pot. You may need to add more water throughout this recipe; do so carefully.

2 Place the dry ts'icháyaý tips in the top pot of the double boiler and pour the syrup over them. Let the syrup gently warm on low heat for 1–2 hours.

3 Remove the syrup from the heat and let cool. Strain out the ts'icháyaý tips and bottle the infused syrup. Store the syrup in the refrigerator and use within 1–2 months.

4 Preheat the oven to 200°F (95°C).

5 Line a cookie sheet with parchment paper. Lay out the ts'icháyaý tips evenly on the sheet and bake them for 30–45 minutes. Extend the time as needed until the ts'icháyaý tips are caramelized. Remove them from the parchment paper and store in a container for snacking!

<u>K</u>wáytsay

kw-ayt-sigh
WESTERN HEMLOCK
Tsuga heterophylla

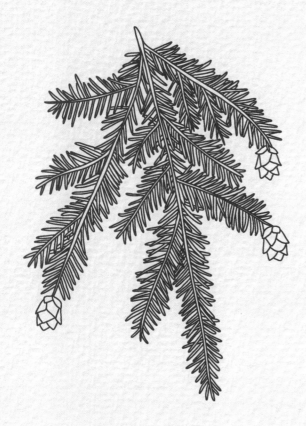

 BUILDING RELATIONSHIPS

The lacy branches of <u>k</u>wáytsay have such a beauty to them. The new growth of the branches (the spring tips) stay light green and tender for weeks. This is a very common tree around the Squamish area. Knowing your tree identification is important here as there is some visual similarity to the yew tree (*Taxus brevifolia*), which is toxic. Though the trees look very different to the trained eye, they could be confused by someone who doesn't have a lot of experience with tree identification. One of the best ways to tell these two trees apart is that <u>k</u>wáytsay has light green needles that are varying lengths and brown twigs, whereas yew trees have dark green needles that are mostly the same length, coming off either side in an even pattern from green twigs. Yew also has fleshy, red berrylike fruit in place of cones. Placing mindful attention toward the sea of green conifers can help you to start developing your skills and abilities to recognize and identify conifer trees more easily until you have built the confidence to start harvesting.

WARNING: *<u>K</u>wáytsay can be mistaken for the toxic yew tree* (Taxus brevifolia). *Be sure to have your tree identification mastered between these two species before harvesting and consuming <u>k</u>wáytsay.*

HABITAT

K̲wáytsay is shade tolerant and can be found growing abundantly at low to mid elevations in moist to dry sites from Oregon to Alaska.

BOTANICAL DESCRIPTION

K̲wáytsay is a tall tree that grows up to 164–196 feet (50–60 m) in height. The crown of the tree is narrow, with a drooping tip. The sweeping branches have delicate, lacy foliage with short, flat needles that are irregular in length. The bark is rough and gray brown, which becomes increasingly furrowed with age. Pollen cones are numerous and very small. Seed cones are also small, approximately 0.8 inch (2 cm) long and egg-shaped.

SUSTAINABLE HARVEST AND TIMING

The new spring tips of the branches are great to harvest through the spring in April and May. Be sure to spread out your harvest. If harvesting the inner bark layer in the spring, make sure to learn from someone who knows how to do this without injuring the tree. Taking the inner bark from smaller branches is a good way not to disturb the bark on the main trunk of the tree.

PLANT GIFTS

K̲wáytsay tips are tender and citrusy and can be eaten from the branch for a burst of vitamin C and electrolytes or infused in water for a delicate, woodsy flavor.

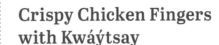

Crispy Chicken Fingers with K̲wáytsay

2 servings

½ pound (225 g) chicken breast
½ cup (120 ml) milk (or nondairy alternative)
2 cups (60 g) cornflakes
2 tablespoons dried k̲wáytsay tips, chopped
½ teaspoon sea salt
½ teaspoon garlic powder
Blueberry and Salal Sauce (page 181), for serving (optional)

1 Preheat the oven to 375°F (190°C).

2 Cut the chicken into even strips and place them in the milk inside a plastic bag or container. Leave the strips fully covered in the milk for 10 minutes.

3 Line a baking tray with parchment paper and set aside.

4 Place the cornflakes into a separate plastic bag and use your hands to crush them into crumbs. The finer the crumbs, the more fully coated the chicken fingers will be. Alternatively, keep the crumbs a bit chunky.

5 Add the chopped k̲wáytsay to the bag of crushed cornflakes, along with salt and garlic powder, and shake, shake, shake.

6 Place the seasoned cornflake crumbs into a shallow bowl.

7 Place one milk-soaked chicken strip at a time into the bowl and roll until the entire strip is well coated in crumbs.

8 Place the coated strips onto the baking tray and bake for 20 minutes, flipping them over after 10 minutes. The chicken should register an internal temperature of 165°F (75°C).

9 Serve with the Blueberry and Salal Sauce, if desired.

X̱ápayay

xe-pie-eye
WESTERN RED CEDAR
Thuja plicata

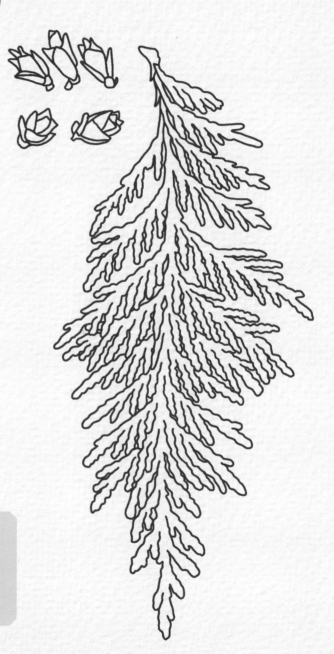

BUILDING RELATIONSHIPS

X̱ápayay is the name for the Western red cedar tree. There are dozens of other Squamish words that are associated with this tree, which is a linguistic indicator of just how culturally significant it is. The inner bark, or sléwey (slaw-eye), is sustainably harvested from living trees to process and utilize in weaving. Each spring I harvest sléwey with my extended family. The harvest brings together all the in-depth knowledge and expertise required to understand when the sap is running, what size tree to harvest from, and what individual trees might yield the longest pulls of bark. I love walking through the forest to find a tree to harvest from while listening to family members talking and harvesting. I can close my eyes and see my children on their first x̱ápayay bark harvest, their tiny hands working their way under the sides of the bark strip, feeling the cold, fresh sap running over their fingers.

WARNING: *Pregnant people and people with kidney disorders should not take x̱ápayay internally. X̱ápayay contains thujone, which in higher concentrations can cause low blood pressure, convulsions, and even death.*

HABITAT

X̱ápay̓ay grows in moist to wet soils, usually in shaded forest sites with rich soils, as well as in boggy woodland, from low to mid elevations. It is found on the Pacific coast from Southeast Alaska through BC, western Washington, and Oregon, reaching into the coastal redwood forests of Northern California.

BOTANICAL DESCRIPTION

X̱ápay̓ay is a large tree that grows up to 197 feet (60 m) in height, with small, drooping branches that have scales instead of needles, giving them a feathery, spray-like appearance. The pollen cones are small and reddish orange, and the seed-bearing cones are approximately 0.4 inch (1 cm) in length and egg-shaped, with eight to twelve scales per cone. The bark is gray to reddish brown and tears off in long, fibrous strands.

SUSTAINABLE HARVEST AND TIMING

Harvesting the inner bark requires much care so as not to injure or overharvest from a single tree. This is a culturally sensitive practice, so I will not give specific instructions for harvesting here. However, my teachings are that a single tree should only be harvested from once, and only a small percentage of the bark should be stripped off. For those who are looking to harvest for cultural reasons, start by reaching out to your (or nearby) Indigenous communities to inquire about local cedar bark-harvesting protocols. Harvest time is in spring when sap is running, which is around May–June in Squamish.

PLANT GIFTS

This tree has been a cultural keystone species for generations upon generations of Indigenous Peoples living within its range. The bark is water-repellent, making the clothing woven with the inner bark water-resistant. The wood, which is light and easily split or carved, has been utilized for everything from canoes for transport to housing in the form of both the planks and posts of longhouses. Western red cedar has strong antibacterial and antifungal properties and can be used topically as an infusion or tincture to treat fungal skin infections.

Stovetop x̱ápay̓ay steam (shared below) can help with congestion if you have a cold. It is also believed to purify and cleanse the air.

Stovetop X̱ápay̓ay Steam

1 use

1–2 fresh-clipped x̱ápay̓ay boughs
Eucalyptus essential oil (optional)

1 Fill a large pot three-quarters full with water.

2 Add the boughs of x̱ápay̓ay.

3 Simmer over low heat on the stovetop. Add water when needed. (Optional: Add a few drops of eucalyptus essential oil to enhance the effect of the steam.)

4 Place your face close to the pot and fan the aromatic steam toward you. Breathe deeply, being careful not to get too close to the steam or hot pot.

5 Pour out the water when you are finished.

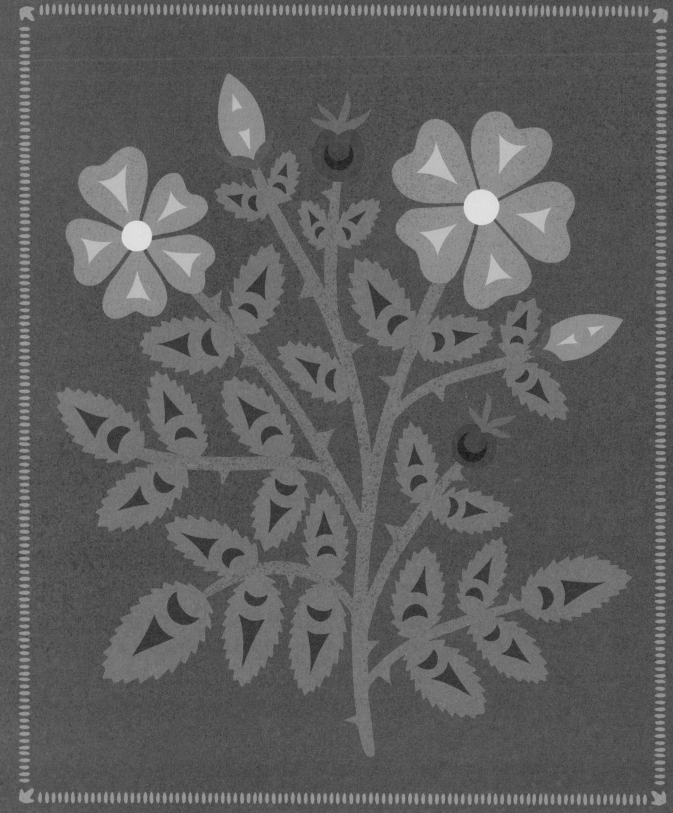

SHRUBS

••• ◀━━●━━▶ •••

K'p'a<u>x</u>w

k-p-ow-x
BEAKED HAZELNUT
Corylus cornuta

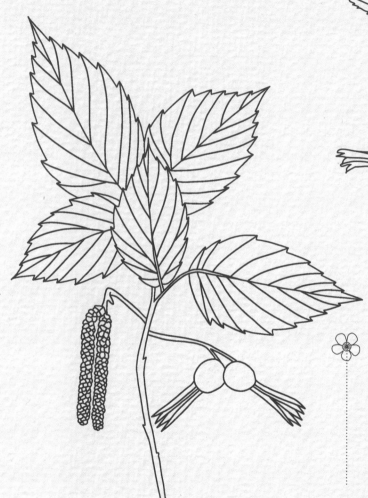

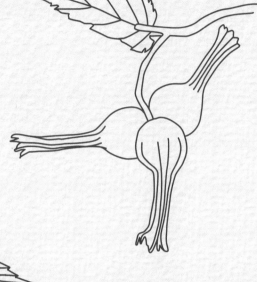

 BUILDING RELATIONSHIPS

K'p'a<u>x</u>w is one of the few nut-bearing trees in the Pacific Northwest. In many Indigenous communities this tree was managed in forest gardens and was, and continues to be, highly regarded as an energy-rich food. My Squamish ancestors picked this food in the fall and stored it in boxes to let it ripen before enjoying it.

WARNING: *If you have nut allergies, do not eat k̲'p'a<u>x</u>w.*

HABITAT

K̲'p'a̲xw grows in open forested sites, thickets, clearings, rocky slopes, and well-drained riparian habitats. It can be found at low to mid elevations across its range, which is concentrated in southern BC and into Washington. It also grows south into Georgia.

BOTANICAL DESCRIPTION

K̲'p'a̲xw is a deciduous shrub that grows up to 3–10 feet (1–3 m) tall with many stems and densely clumped, moderately hairy twigs. K̲'p'a̲xw spreads by suckers. The leaves are oval with a heart-shaped base, sharp tip, and toothed margins. They measure 1.6–4 inches (4–10 cm) long, are green (paler underneath than on top), and turn yellow in the fall. The male catkins appear before the leaves in the spring; the female catkins are small with distinct, protruding red stigmas. The fruit is an edible nut that is 0.6 inch (1.5 cm) long and grows in bunches of three to four at the ends of the branches in a light-green husk. The husk is covered with stiff prickly hairs that project beyond the nut into the beak that gives it its English name. Two varieties occur in BC.

SUSTAINABLE HARVEST AND TIMING

The nuts of k̲'p'a̲xw are ready for harvest in the late summer, which in the Squamish region would be late August or early September. It is advisable to wear gloves to harvest the nuts as they have hairs on the outer husk that can irritate your fingers. The nuts can be husked while you harvest, or after a few days of drying. K̲'p'a̲xw trees are not widely available in many areas of BC, so historically these nuts would have been traded. Because of this last point, in addition to the nuts being a prized food for wildlife, you will want to spread out your harvest and not take too many from one tree.

PLANT GIFTS

The nuts of k̲'p'a̲xw are rich in carbohydrates, fats, and proteins, and are a bit of a rarity as there is not an abundance of nut-bearing shrubs or trees in the Squamish area. However, the fruit can be planted out and germinated to produce more trees. Store the nuts in a cool, dry place for up to twelve months.

K̲'p'a̲xw Dairy-Free Ice Cream

4 cups (560 g)

2 tablespoons k̲'p'a̲xw
4 frozen bananas
2 tablespoons vanilla extract
1 teaspoon ground cinnamon

1   Toast the k̲'p'a̲xw in a dry skillet over low heat until lightly browned, which will take around 10–15 minutes. Make sure that the k̲'p'a̲xw are spread out evenly in the pan. Let the k̲'p'a̲xw cool and roughly chop.

2   Blend all the ingredients together in a food processor or blender until smooth.

3   Store the ice cream in an airtight container in the freezer for up to 3 months.

Make ice cream sandwiches with your favorite cookies!

Ts'ḵw'uḿáý

ts-oh-kw-om-eye

BLACKCAP

Rubus leucodermis

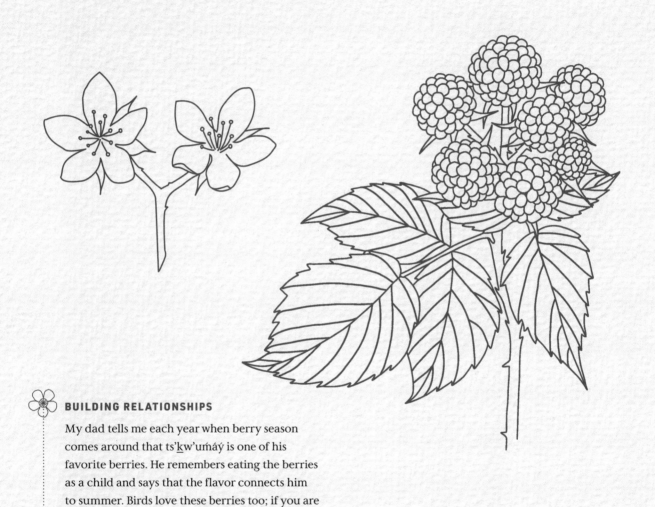

BUILDING RELATIONSHIPS

My dad tells me each year when berry season comes around that ts'ḵw'uḿáý is one of his favorite berries. He remembers eating the berries as a child and says that the flavor connects him to summer. Birds love these berries too; if you are planting them in a garden setting, you might place them in a hedgerow along your fence so birds are able to access some of the berries. This plant thrives in full sun and moisture, so it is a great one for your garden.

HABITAT

Ts'ḵw'uṁáý occurs in dry to moist thickets, rocky slopes, clearings, and open forests at low to mid elevations. It is common in southwestern BC and extends south to California.

BOTANICAL DESCRIPTION

Ts'ḵw'uṁáý is a deciduous shrub that grows 3–7 feet (1–2 m) tall. The stems have curved, flattened prickles and are covered with a whitish bloom. The compound leaves have three to five leaflets, and are green above and white woolly beneath, with saw-toothed edges. Flowers are whitish to pink and are 0.8–1.2 inches (2–3 cm) across. The reddish-purple to black raspberries grow in clusters of two to ten.

SUSTAINABLE HARVEST AND TIMING

The spring shoots come out in April in the Pacific Northwest and can be harvested sparingly across ts'ḵw'uṁáý plants. These shoots are the new spring growth, so if you harvest them, be mindful of whether you are thinning out the bush. The berries ripen in the summer months and are a favorite for birds and other wildlife. Spread out your harvest to be mindful of other non-human life that rely on the berries. Or, better yet, grow them in your garden!

PLANT GIFTS

The early spring shoots of ts'ḵw'uṁáý are high in vitamin C and can be peeled and eaten fresh or cooked, like asparagus. The berries are wonderful fresh or can be dried into cakes or fruit leather. They are rich in anthocyanins and antioxidants, which make them very good for supporting overall health. A mild tea can be made from the leaves that is rich in vitamin C.

Ts'ḵw'uṁáý Berry Cobbler

6–8 servings

Berry Filling

4 cups (560 g) fresh or frozen ts'ḵw'uṁáý berries (you can mix with other summer berries)
½ lemon, juiced (about ⅛ cup, or 30 ml)
1 teaspoon vanilla extract
¼ cup (30 g) all-purpose flour or almond flour
1 tablespoon brown sugar or maple syrup (optional)

Topping

1 cup (90 g) rolled oats
1¼ cups (146 g) crushed walnuts or pecans
¼ teaspoon ground cinnamon
1 cup (125 g) + 2 tablespoons all-purpose flour or almond flour
2 tablespoons extra-virgin coconut oil, melted and cooled
½ cup (110 g or 120 ml) brown sugar or maple syrup
½ teaspoon vanilla extract
Dairy or nondairy ice cream of choice, for serving

1 Preheat the oven to 350°F (175°C) and take out a round baking dish; about 8–9 inches (20–23 cm) works great!

2 In a medium bowl, mix all the ingredients for the berry filling.

3 In a separate, large bowl, mix all the ingredients for the cobbler topping.

4 Pour the berry filling into the baking dish and spread evenly.

5 Add the cobbler topping and cover the berries completely.

6 Bake the cobbler in the oven for 45–50 minutes, or until the top is golden or slightly browned.

7 Allow the cobbler to cool for about 10 minutes, then serve, topped with some ice cream!

Xwíxwikw'ay, Iẏálk̲paẏ

xw-eh-xw-ikw-eye ay-all-k-p-eye

BLUEBERRY

Vaccinium ovalifolium, V. alaskaense

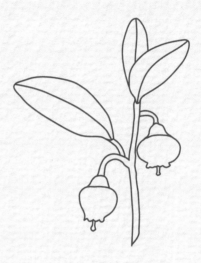

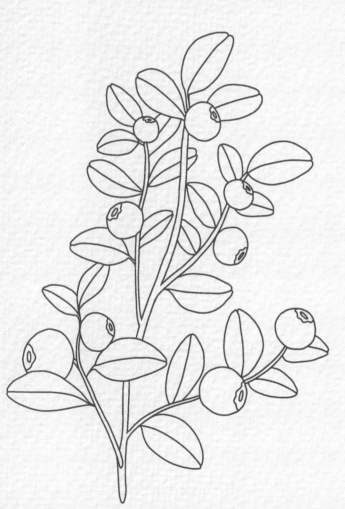

 BUILDING RELATIONSHIPS

Each fall I go up into the subalpine meadows in Squamish Territory with my family to pick alpine xwíxwikw'ay, also known as iẏálk̲paẏ. I love getting into higher elevations, being closer to the mountains, smelling the fir pitch on the breeze, and seeing the heathers underfoot as we make our way with care through the meadows and hillsides to pick the berries. Autumn's beautiful yellow, red, and orange leaves paint the landscape. My children eat berries while I try to fill my basket with the delicious and nutritious berries, which I'll bring home to store in the freezer and add to our morning oatmeal throughout the winter months. I enjoy reflecting on the knowledge that my Squamish ancestors picked these same foods in the same subalpine meadows where I go with my children.

HABITAT

Xwíxwikw'ay generally grows in moist coniferous forests, forest edges, and around bogs and subalpine thickets. It grows as a shrub that forms dense patches from low to high elevations. Xwíxwikw'ay is common in central and southern BC and can be found from Alaska and the southern Yukon and is disjunct in Ontario, Newfoundland, and Nova Scotia. It grows south to Oregon and Montana. The habitat may vary slightly based on what edible species of berry you are harvesting.

BOTANICAL DESCRIPTION

Xwíxwikw'ay leaves are thin and oval-shaped and range from green to reddish in color. The flowers are small, pink, and bell-shaped. The berries range from dark purple to blue in color.

SUSTAINABLE HARVEST AND TIMING

Don't forget that bears love and rely on xwíxwikw'ay and other wild berries! This means you should take care when you are out harvesting and ensure you make noise to let your presence be known. Don't overharvest from a single bush or area. Spread out your harvest. The berries can be harvested in late August through September when they are ripe, and the leaves can be harvested throughout the growing season.

PLANT GIFTS

This plant is one that connects directly to our health and helps us to build relationships with the subalpine environments where Indigenous Peoples have traveled seasonally for thousands of years to harvest key food and medicine plants. The berries in particular are a local superfood! They are very high in antioxidants and can help improve overall health when consumed regularly. These antioxidants are helpful in maintaining heart health and can reduce chronic inflammation. Additionally, a tea made from the leaves can help stabilize blood sugars and settle upset stomachs.

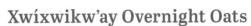

Xwíxwikw'ay Overnight Oats

4 servings

NOTE: *This recipe is made in a slow cooker.*

Butter or oil of your choosing (coconut or vegetable oil works well), for greasing
1–2 cups (145–290 g) xwíxwikw'ay, fresh or frozen
1 cup (155 g) uncooked steel-cut oats (regular rolled oats can be substituted)
1½ cups (360 ml) milk or nondairy alternative like almond, coconut, or oat milk
1½ cups (360 ml) water
1 teaspoon ground cinnamon
2 tablespoons brown sugar (substitute maple syrup or other sweetener)
1 teaspoon vanilla extract
¼ teaspoon salt
1½ tablespoons butter, cut into 5–6 pieces (optional)
1 tablespoon ground flaxseed or chia seed (optional)
* Optional garnishes: chopped nuts, shredded coconut, maple syrup, milk, or nondairy alternative of your choosing

1 Coat the inside of a slow cooker with butter or oil.

2 Add all the ingredients to the slow cooker; stir and cover.

3 Cook on low for approximately 7 hours (time may vary based on your slow cooker).

4 Wake up and serve the oatmeal warm from the pot, garnish as desired, and enjoy!

5 Store leftovers in the fridge overnight to eat the next day, or freeze for later.

<u>K</u>wemchúḷs

kwem-ch-oh-l-s

BOG CRANBERRY

Vaccinium oxycoccos,
V. vitis-idaea

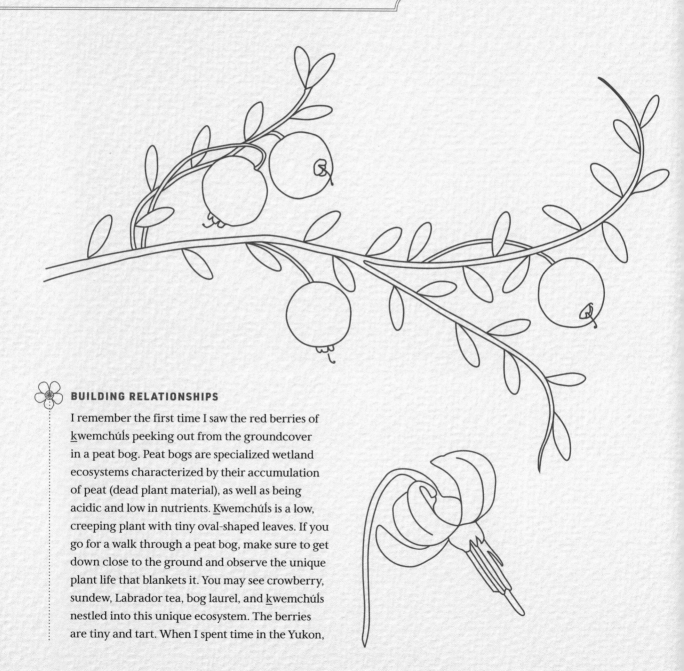

🌸 **BUILDING RELATIONSHIPS**

I remember the first time I saw the red berries of
<u>k</u>wemchúḷs peeking out from the groundcover
in a peat bog. Peat bogs are specialized wetland
ecosystems characterized by their accumulation
of peat (dead plant material), as well as being
acidic and low in nutrients. <u>K</u>wemchúḷs is a low,
creeping plant with tiny oval-shaped leaves. If you
go for a walk through a peat bog, make sure to get
down close to the ground and observe the unique
plant life that blankets it. You may see crowberry,
sundew, Labrador tea, bog laurel, and <u>k</u>wemchúḷs
nestled into this unique ecosystem. The berries
are tiny and tart. When I spent time in the Yukon,

the ground was covered with lowbush cranberry (*Vaccinium vitis-idaea*), a relative of k̲wemchúĺs; its deep purple-red berries carry a burst of vitamin C and a sweet, tangy, delicious flavor. As each fall approached in the Yukon, we'd head out with baskets in hand and spend hours picking the tiny berries from between the caribou lichen and crowberry. Crouching down, we observed the beauty of the boreal botanical groundcover as we searched for the little pops of color that signaled the next cranberry patch.

HABITAT

K̲wemchúĺs grows in bogs and fens at low to mid elevations, and sometimes in wet subalpine meadows. It is frequent throughout BC, north to Alaska and the Yukon, and south to Oregon. Both *V. oxycoccos* and *V. vitis-idaea* are circumboreal. *V. vitis-idaea* grows in bogs, peaty tundra, and wet to dry, mossy forests, from low to high elevations.

BOTANICAL DESCRIPTION

K̲wemchúĺs is a small, creeping shrub with slender, vinelike stems that are 6–20 inches (15–51 cm) long. It has small evergreen leaves that are 0.08–0.4 inch (2–10 mm) long, alternate, egg-shaped to elliptic, pointy-tipped and leathery. The leaves are shiny on the upper surface and grayish beneath, with margins rolled under. Flowers are deep pink and shaped like mini shooting star flowers (*Dodecatheon* spp.), with petals angled up and long-stalked in clusters of one to three. Berries are pale pink to dark red in color and 0.2–0.5 inch (5–12 mm) wide. *V. vitis-idaea* also has small evergreen leaves that are egg-shaped, but with rounded tips and tiny brown dots on the underside. It has clusters of short-stalked, white to pink, bell-shaped flowers and red berries.

SUSTAINABLE HARVEST AND TIMING

K̲wemchúĺs is harvested in the fall when the berries are ripe. They start to sweeten with overnight frosts. Ensure you are harvesting from an area where the k̲wemchúĺs is plentiful. Be sure to leave some for the non-human life that rely on them and do not overharvest an area. Some years are better k̲wemchúĺs years than others. Get to know your harvesting areas and you can go back year after year to harvest these little red gems.

PLANT GIFTS

K̲wemchúĺs is rich in vitamin C. The berries and leaves have historically been used to support bladder and urinary tract health. The berries are rich in antioxidants, making them a wonderful food that supports overall health and immunity. They freeze well and can be used to make homemade juice or the cranberry sauce included here.

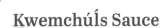

K̲wemchúĺs Sauce

2 cups (474 ml)

2–3 cups (190–285 g) k̲wemchúĺs
⅔ cup (160 ml) fresh-squeezed orange juice
½–1 cup (100–200 g) sugar (to taste)
1 tablespoon orange zest (optional)

1   Add all the ingredients to a medium saucepan.

2   Stir continuously over medium heat for 10 minutes.

3   Carefully pour the sauce into bowls and place in the fridge to set for at least 2–3 hours for a firmer sauce.

Ch'átyaý

ch-awt-ee-eye
DEVIL'S CLUB
Oplopanax horridus

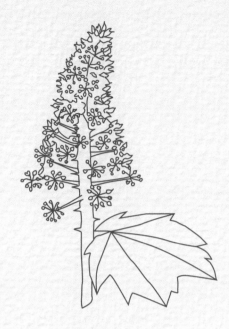

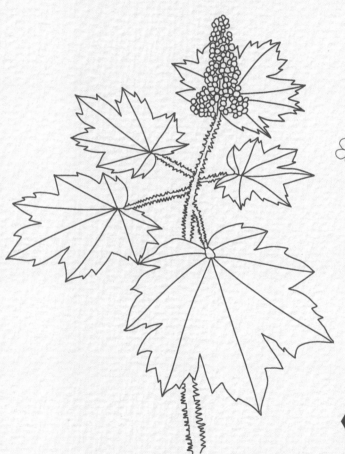

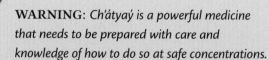

BUILDING RELATIONSHIPS

Ch'átyaý is one of the most culturally and spiritually important plants in Squamish Territory and across its range in general. Each spring when the forests start to awaken, the scent of ch'átyaý signals its presence. Later in the season, the leaves will grow large and contribute to the cacophony of green that characterizes temperate rainforests in the late spring and throughout the summer. I go out with family and community members to harvest this plant each season, and I always process some bark to give back to the community for health or ceremonial uses.

WARNING: *Ch'átyaý is a powerful medicine that needs to be prepared with care and knowledge of how to do so at safe concentrations. Please do not consume this plant without expert guidance from someone who holds cultural knowledge of ch'átyaý medicine.*

HABITAT

Ch'átyaý grows at low to mid elevations in moist to wet, usually somewhat open forests, and particularly in wet but well-drained river terraces, sloping seepage sites, gullies, and along streams. It seems to require the cool humid microclimate of moist forests, and suffers when the forest cover is removed. Ch'átyaý grows from Alaska along the Pacific Northwest coast down into Washington, Oregon, and Northern California.

BOTANICAL DESCRIPTION

Ch'átyaý is an erect-to-sprawling plant that grows to 3–10 feet (1–3 m) high and mostly unbranched. The stems, branches, and underside of the leaves are covered in large spines up to 0.4 inch (1 cm) long. The maple-shaped leaves are large, growing up to 14 inches (35 cm) across. The small, greenish-white flowers grow in compact, pyramid-shaped clusters atop the stems, as do the bright red berries.

SUSTAINABLE HARVEST AND TIMING

I suggest asking yourself, "Should I harvest this plant?" Consider: Is ch'átyaý part of your cultural heritage? Do you know how abundant ch'átyaý is in the region you live in? Do you have enough knowledge and experience to harvest ch'átyaý safely? If you do decide to harvest, and you've gotten permission from either your own Indigenous community or the local Indigenous community, then you will need to survey the regions where ch'átyaý grows to be sure you harvest from a place where the plant is thriving. Process the stalk while it is fresh. This includes carefully scraping off all the spines and then shaving the green layer of the bark into strips so it is ready to dry in a basket over the next three to four days. Because this plant can root out from its nodes, I clip off the top of the plant below one of the nodes and replant it into the ground.

PLANT GIFTS

Ch'átyaý is a wonderful topical medicine that is anti-inflammatory and antibacterial. The bark can be used sparingly to steep as a tea. The flavor is green, woodsy, and fresh. You need to take care when ingesting this plant as it is very potent. I recommend you learn from someone who knows how to prepare it safely before you ingest it.

Ch'átyaý-Infused Oil
1 quart (1 L)

1 cup (20 g) dried ch'átyaý bark
1 quart (1 L) carrier oil (sunflower, jojoba, and olive oils are all great options)

1　Pour water in the bottom pot of a double boiler, being careful not to have the water touching the bottom of the top pot, and place the top pot over it.

2　Fill the top pot with oil and place the dried bark in the oil.

3　Simmer the oil over medium heat for 2–4 hours, adding water to the bottom pot to make sure it does not evaporate completely.

4　Remove the double boiler from the heat and let it cool to room temperature.

5　Carefully lift the top pot and wipe the outside with a towel to remove any condensation.

6　Strain the oil through cheesecloth into a clean, dry 1-quart (1-L) jar.

7　Let the oil cool completely before you place a lid on the jar and store it in the fridge for later use as a body or bath oil.

Kwú7kwuwel̓s

kwoh-kwoh-wel-s
HIGHBUSH CRANBERRY
Viburnum edule

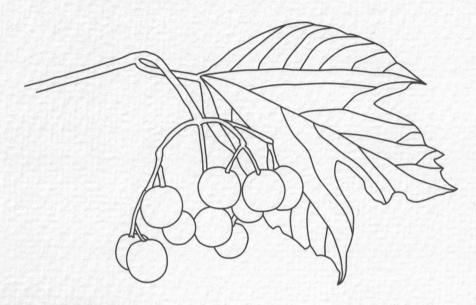

BUILDING RELATIONSHIPS

I first learned about kwú7kwuwel̓s when I was living in Tahltan territory in northern BC. I kept hearing about a plant called highbush cranberry that wasn't actually a cranberry, and I was intrigued. Because of how abundant it is in that area, along with how the fruit grows in dense clusters, this was an easy harvest once I found large stands of kwú7kwuwel̓s to harvest from.

HABITAT

Kwú7kwuwel̓s grows in wet to moist sites, including streambanks, swamps, and forests at low elevations. Kwú7kwuwel̓s is found growing frequently throughout BC, north to Alaska and the Yukon, and south to Oregon.

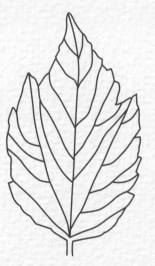

BOTANICAL DESCRIPTION

Kwú7kwuwel̓s is a deciduous shrub that spreads from rhizomes and stands 3–10 feet (1–3 m) tall, with smooth bark that is reddish to gray in color. The leaves are opposite, stalked, shallowly three-lobed (with some that are unlobed), jaggedly toothed, and hairy underneath, especially along the veins. The leaves turn crimson in the fall. Kwú7kwuwel̓s has small, compact clusters of a few to several flowers that are 0.1–0.4 inch (0.3–1 cm) across. Fruits are clusters of round red or orange berrylike structures that are 0.3–0.6 inch (0.8–1.5 cm) across, each with a single, large, flattened stone.

SUSTAINABLE HARVEST AND TIMING

The fruit of kwú7kwuwel̓s is ready to harvest in late August and into September. Some people believe the fruit is sweeter after the first frost. Be mindful to look for a large stand of kwú7kwuwel̓s before harvesting, and be sure to leave at least half the fruit on each bush for wildlife to enjoy.

PLANT GIFTS

Kwú7kwuwel̓s is rich in vitamins A and C, and the juice has been used to support urinary tract health and lower blood sugar. The bark is a strong antispasmodic. Another common name for this plant is crampbark because an infusion of the dried bark can help with muscle cramps. The fruit is strongly scented and has a large seed that needs to be removed before consuming, so lends itself well to juices and jelly.

Kwú7kwuwel̓s Jelly

approximately 3 cups (1020 g)

5 cups (500 g) kwú7kwuwel̓s
3 cups (720 ml) water
1 package (57 g) of powdered pectin
4 cups (800 g) sugar
3 tablespoons fresh-squeezed lemon juice

1   Place the kwú7kwuwel̓s and water in a large pot. Bring to a boil, then boil for 10 minutes. Gently crush the berries as they begin to soften.

2   Let the berries cool. Strain them through cheesecloth.

3   Measure out 4½ cups (1.1 L) of the juice, pour into the pot, and add the pectin. Place the pot onto the stovetop and heat the mixture to a boil, stirring nonstop.

4   Pour in the sugar and lemon juice and stir the mixture until dissolved.

5   Bring the heat up again and boil for 1 minute without stirring. Remove the pot from the heat and use a spoon to scoop off and discard foam that may have formed on the surface.

6   Place the jelly in clean, hot canning jars. Wipe the tops of the jars to remove any spillage and cover with the lids.

7   Seal the lids on the jars in a hot-water bath for 10 minutes. If any lids do not seal, refrigerate and use within 3 weeks.

    If for some reason the jelly does not set, you can use it as a syrup to add to sparkling water as a refreshing drink.

Mákwam

m-aw-kw-am

LABRADOR TEA

Rhododendron groenlandicum

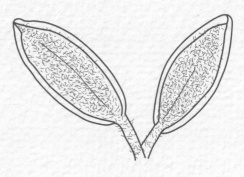

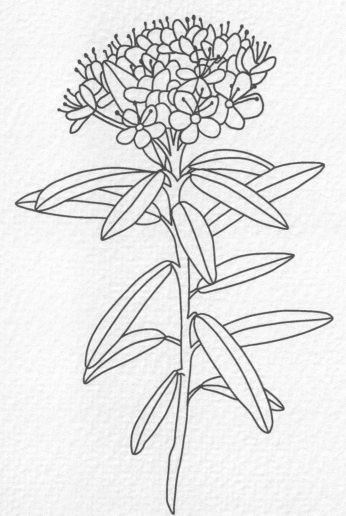

BUILDING RELATIONSHIPS

Mákwam is a strong plant medicine and is one of the first plants I learned about. I remember walking through a bog trail on the west side of Vancouver Island in Tla-o-qui-aht territory and seeing mákwam growing. I learned how to differentiate it from the poisonous bog laurel (*Kalmia microphylla*) that grows beside it. Mákwam has a distinct woolly underside to the leaf, among other key features. This leaf was made into a tea by my Squamish relatives and ancestors and was used to ease symptoms of tuberculosis.

WARNING: *If you are making tea, pour the boiling water over the leaves and steep them; boiling them in water will result in a concentrated decoction that can be harmful. Please also refer to the note above about mákwam's poisonous lookalike, the bog laurel (Kalmia microphylla).*

HABITAT

Mákwam grows in peat bogs, boggy forests, and along lake shores at low to mid elevations. It thrives in wet, acidic peatlands, and also does well in dry forests, especially boreal forests, in nutrient-poor soils. Mákwam is common along the coast from Alaska to Oregon, and inland across the continent to northeast North America and Greenland.

BOTANICAL DESCRIPTION

Mákwam is a low-spreading to upright, branched shrub that usually grows 0.98–3 feet (0.3–1 m) tall, with leathery, evergreen, often drooping leaves that alternate up the stem. Leaves are lance-shaped to oblong and 0.8–2 inches (2–5 cm) long, with rolled-under margins. The upper leaf surface is deep green and the leaf underside has a dense rust-colored or yellowish soft-hairy surface. The small white flowers are numerous in compact, umbrella-like clusters; each flower has five petals. Numerous small seeds are produced in dry, egg-shaped capsules.

SUSTAINABLE HARVEST AND TIMING

Mákwam leaves can be harvested from spring until the early fall and should be harvested sparingly from individual plants. Only harvest if the overall stand of the plants is healthy and plentiful.

PLANT GIFTS

Mákwam leaves are rich in vitamin C and are a plant medicine with a long history of treating respiratory ailments. The leaves are anti-inflammatory and can be used topically to calm skin and help resolve breakouts. If ingesting mákwam, you need to take care not to concentrate the plant too much.

Mákwam Facial Clay

1½ cups (140 g)

1 teaspoon mákwam leaf
1 teaspoon yarrow leaf
½ cup (40 g) white kaolin clay
½ cup (40 g) green clay or bentonite clay
½ cup (60 g) finely ground oats
¼ teaspoon activated charcoal

1   Use a blender or coffee grinder to crush the mákwam and yarrow leaves into a powder. Sift the powder through a fine-mesh sieve to remove large bits.

2   Add all the remaining ingredients together in a dry, clean bowl and, using a whisk, mix well to break up any clumps and ensure that the ingredients are all well distributed throughout the powder.

3   Use a metal funnel to pour the powder mixture into either one large glass jar or a set of smaller jars. If you don't have a metal funnel, you can use a piece of paper rolled up into a cone to help pour the powder into the jars.

4   Using a teaspoon amount in the palm of your hand, add enough water to make a paste. Apply the paste to your face and either leave on as a face mask for 10–15 minutes or gently exfoliate. Rinse off the facial clay with warm water.

Kálxaý

k-aw-l-x-eye
OCEAN SPRAY
Holodiscus discolor

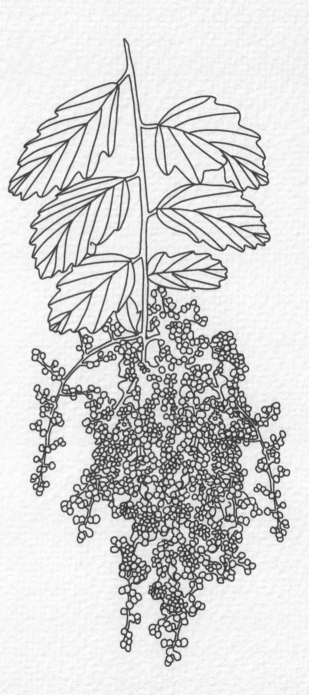

BUILDING RELATIONSHIPS

My father is a wood carver; he recalls, as a child, using kálxaý to make bows because it had the flexibility and strength for the job. I love being able to walk through the natural world and see the interrelationships between people and plants. Knowing the ways that kálxaý wood was utilized by my ancestors brings a new depth of meaning to enjoying the flowering season where the ample cream-colored flowers hang down and bloom in bunches. Layering stories on top of lived land-based experiences enriches my knowledge of how I as a Squamish person am intertwined with the ecosystem in my homelands.

HABITAT

Kálxaý grows in dry to mesic open forests, edges, and thickets, as well as on coastal bluffs and rocky slopes. It also often grows in open, disturbed areas, such as logged or burned areas and roadsides. Its growing range extends from southern BC to Southern California, and east to the Rockies.

BOTANICAL DESCRIPTION

Ḵálx̱aý is a shrub that grows to 2.5 feet (0.8 m) tall and can be recognized by its alternate, oval-to-triangular leaves with margins that are lobed or coarsely and doubly toothed. The green upper surface of the leaves can be smooth or covered in coarse hair; the paler undersurface is strongly veined and covered in soft hairs. Ḵálx̱aý flowers are white to cream in color with drooping, lilac-like clusters.

SUSTAINABLE HARVEST AND TIMING

The branches of ḵálx̱aý can be harvested year-round, but because you are taking a limb from the plant, be sure to select the branch carefully. Before cutting the branch, find the right thickness and straightness for the job. If you are making roasting sticks, you want a branch that is about 1 inch (2.5 cm) thick, whereas if you are making a digging stick, you want a branch or main trunk of the shrub that is approximately 4–5 inches (10–13 cm) thick.

PLANT GIFTS

Ḵálx̱aý is an important technology plant that has been used to create many different implements, including needles, arrows, digging sticks, and more. Its tensile strength and ability to fire-harden lend itself well to these applications. The Squamish name ḵálx̱aý translates directly to "digging-stick-bush"; this refers to a sḵalx̱ or a traditional digging stick that was used in Squamish to dig up precious root foods and clams. I have utilized digging sticks to harvest root vegetables, as there is no other harvesting tool that is more accurate and that causes the least amount of disturbance to surrounding plant roots. These sticks are traditionally very narrow, with a pointed tip and a rounded handle to maximize the accuracy of digging out small roots. I have also had the opportunity to attend outdoor cooking events in WSÁNEĆ territory with elder and knowledge holder Earl Claxton Jr., and he is the one who taught me about cooking seafood on ḵálx̱aý skewers, as in the recipe below. Earl says that this method of cooking clams actually sweetens the meat and gives them a delicious, smokey flavor!

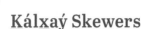

Ḵálx̱aý Skewers
10–15 servings

10–15 small ḵálx̱aý branches
Seafood (such as clams out of the shell, shrimp, or scallops) or chopped vegetables (such as peppers, onions, tomatoes, or other veggies of your choice). Get creative!

NOTE: *Handle this recipe with caution. Be very careful when around open flames and keep a fire-extinguishing source nearby.*

1   Clean off any side branches and outer bark from the ḵálx̱aý branches with a knife.

2   Use the knife to carefully sharpen one end.

3   For extra strength, try quickly running the skewers through the flames of an open fire ahead of time.

4   Spear your favorite seafood or veggies on the ḵálx̱aý skewers. Place around the open fire by sticking the bottom of each skewer into the sand or dirt close to the fire, or soak the skewers in water prior to roasting on a barbecue.

5   After cooking, remove the food from the skewers and place in a bowl to keep it clean from the surrounding dirt or sand.

Sts'iwḵ'

sts-ew-k

RED ELDERBERRY AND BLUE ELDERBERRY

Sambucus racemosa, S. cerulea

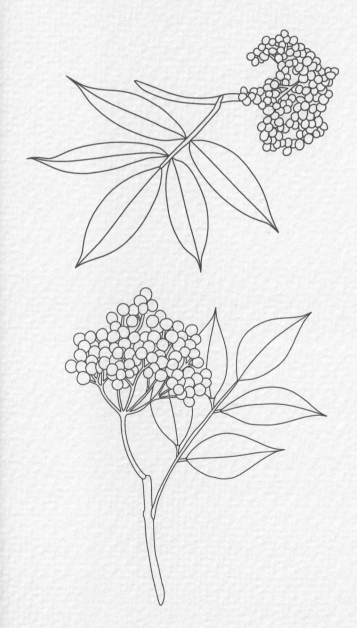

BUILDING RELATIONSHIPS

Sts'iwḵ' is a plant whose reputation precedes it. I have many friends and family members that utilize sts'iwḵ' yearly to support their health. Red elderberry (*Sambucus racemosa*) grows commonly in the Squamish region, although the name sts'iwḵ' refers to both red and blue elderberry. Elderberry species need to be processed carefully as they contain cyanide-producing glycosides—compounds that, in larger amounts, can cause cyanide poisoning. The good news is that, when the berries of both red and blue elderberry are removed from the stems and leaves and cooked, they are safe to use in recipes and to consume to support health and wellness.

HABITAT

Sts'iwḵ' grows in moist sites, including along stream banks, depressions, and open forest clearings. Red elderberry grows extensively from Alaska all along the coast of the Pacific Northwest. Blue elderberry is common in southern BC and grows south to California.

WARNING: *The berries of blue and red elderberry plants are never eaten fresh because of these cyanide-producing glycosides. Do not consume the leaves or stems of this plant, as the toxin is more concentrated in those parts.*

BOTANICAL DESCRIPTION

Sts'iw<u>k</u>' is a large deciduous shrub that grows upward to 3–20 feet (1–6 m) tall, with thick twigs that are soft and contain pith. The bark is a dark reddish brown with small bumps. The large, compound, and pinnately divided leaves grow opposite, and have five to seven elliptic to lanceolate leaflets that are usually somewhat hairy beneath. The small, cream-colored red elderberry flowers grow numerously in cone-shaped clusters that are 1.6–4 inches (4–10 cm) long. Blue elderberry flowers grow in flat-topped clusters and measure up to 8 inches (20 cm) in diameter. The fruits are circular, berrylike, and shiny. They are red or purplish black in color and measure 0.2–0.24 inch (5–6 mm) across. Occasionally, the blue elderberry has a white powdery appearance on the outside of the berries.

SUSTAINABLE HARVEST AND TIMING

Red elderberries are prolific in my region, so it is easy to spread the harvest across different stands. Wildlife love the fruit, so be sure to leave enough on the plant for non-human life. If blue elderberry is harder to find in your region (as it is in mine), it makes an ideal species to plant in your garden. The flowers can be harvested in May in Squamish, but it will vary depending on your region. The berries of both red and blue elderberry ripen in the mid to late summer in July and early August.

PLANT GIFTS

Sts'iw<u>k</u>' carries many gifts. The tiny flowers make a delicious spring elixir when prepared carefully. Blue elderberries are also highly antioxidant and antiviral, which makes any concentrates very good for supporting health, especially through cold and flu season.

Sts'iw<u>k</u>' Blossom Cordial

1 quart (1 L)

2 cups (56 g) sts'iw<u>k</u>' flower heads with stems removed (approximately 15–20 flower heads)
2 lemons, zested and juiced (approximately ½ cup, or 120 ml)
1 teaspoon citric acid
4 cups (800 g) sugar
1 quart (1 L) water

1   Use clippers or scissors to trim the sts'iw<u>k</u>' flowers off of the stalks into a large bowl. The stems are toxic so be sure to remove as many of them from the flowers as you can. A few small pieces of stem will not be enough to hurt you, but you want to be as thorough as possible. This step takes time, but it is worth it!

2   Zest and juice the lemons. Add the zest, citric acid, and lemon juice to another bowl.

3   In a large pot over medium heat, add the sugar and water and bring to a boil, stirring to help the sugar dissolve. Once it has been dissolved, turn off the heat and let the syrup cool to room temperature. Pour the syrup over the flowers, add the lemon mix, and stir to combine.

4   Cover the bowl with cheesecloth and leave it for 48 hours in the fridge.

5   After 48 hours, strain the cordial through a fine-mesh sieve lined with cheesecloth into a clean bottle or jar. Store in the fridge and use within 1–2 weeks.

6   Add 1–3 tablespoons of the cordial into a glass and add sparkling water for a refreshing treat!

Skw'ekwchsáy

s-kw-ak-ch-s-eye
RED HUCKLEBERRY
Vaccinium parvifolium

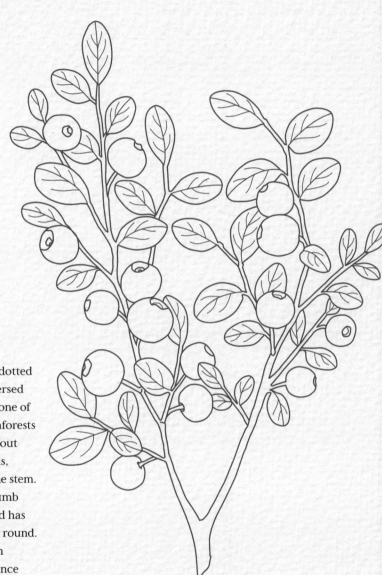

BUILDING RELATIONSHIPS

The lacy branches of skw'ekwchsáy, when dotted
with the bright orange-red berries interspersed
between the small oval-shaped leaves, are one of
the most beautiful sights in the coastal rainforests
where they grow. One of the first things about
identifying skw'ekwchsáy that I tell my kids,
along with the students I teach, is to feel the stem.
Roll it between your pointer finger and thumb
and you will feel that the stem is square and has
distinct edges instead of being smooth and round.
It is these kinds of distinct features that can
support building relationships and confidence
with plant identification over time.

HABITAT

Skw'ekwchsáy occurs in dry to moist forests, forest openings and edges, and frequently on nurse logs, which are fallen and decaying logs that provide habitat, moisture, and nutrients to seedlings as the logs break down over time. Skw'ekwchsáy is found along the Pacific coast from southeast Alaska to central California, mostly in the lowland forests west of the Cascades in BC, Washington, and Oregon, as well as the California coast and the Sierra Nevadas.

BOTANICAL DESCRIPTION

Skw'ekwchsáy is a deciduous shrub that grows typically 3–10 feet (1–3 m) tall, with green, strongly angled branches. Leaves are alternate and oval-shaped and approximately 0.4–1.2 inches (1–3 cm) in length. Skw'ekwchsáy is part of the *Vaccinium* genus, which is a group of woody plants that all have urn- or bell-shaped flowers and produce berries. The berries are bright orangey red, round, and about 0.4 inch (1 cm) across.

SUSTAINABLE HARVEST AND TIMING

The plant blooms in April–June and the fruit ripens in July–August. The leaves of the plant can be harvested year-round and dried for tea. The fruit can be harvested while remembering the other life that rely on the berries, including bears, birds, and other wildlife.

PLANT GIFTS

The leaves of skw'ekwchsáy can be made into a tea to help with bladder and urinary tract health. In fact, a strong infusion of the roots was part of a stomach medicine utilized by my Squamish ancestors. The berries are rich in vitamin C and antioxidants. Skw'ekwchsáy is one type of huckleberry found in this region, but huckleberries overall are known to be one of the few fruits that don't raise blood sugar. This is because they have compounds that can help lower blood sugar, which counteract the sugar in the fruit.

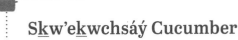

Skw'ekwchsáy Cucumber Salad

1–2 servings

1 cup (104 g) cucumber
1 cup (245 g) tomatoes
½ cup (74 g) skw'ekwchsáy
1 teaspoon lemon juice
1 teaspoon balsamic vinegar
¼ teaspoon sea salt
½ cup (57 g) chopped feta cheese (optional)
Nuts or seeds (optional)

1 Chop the cucumber and tomatoes into small pieces and place them in a small bowl.

2 Add in the fresh skw'ekwchsáy, lemon juice, balsamic vinegar, and salt and gently mix together with a fork. Sprinkle the feta cheese on top if using.

3 To boost the protein content, add in any nuts or seeds you like. Toast them for an extra treat!

4 Serve as a side to any main meal, for lunch, as a quick on-the-go afternoon pick-me-up, or as a snack.

Ḵwiⅼayus

kw-ill-eye-os

RED-FLOWERING CURRANT

Ribes sanguineum

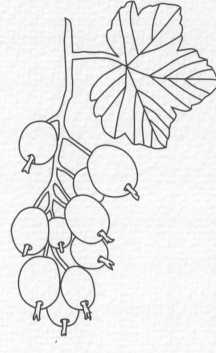

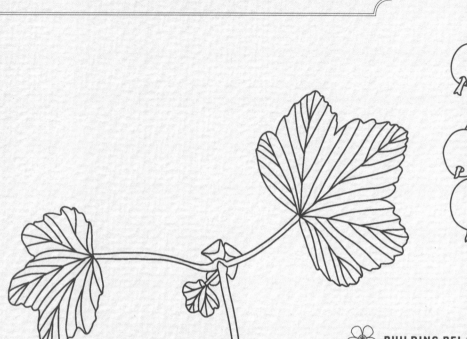

BUILDING RELATIONSHIPS

The cascading fuchsia-colored blooms of ḵwiⅼayus are a sight to behold! There is no other color quite like that of this gorgeous flower. When you happen upon this plant, stop and breathe in the floral and slightly spiced scent. I find connecting to scents is a wonderful way to engage in your natural surroundings and start to build your relationships with the seasonality of the plants that grow around you. These flowers are important for hummingbirds (they particularly draw the migrating rufous hummingbird) as well as butterfly larvae, which use the leaves for food. The berries are edible, though not very flavorful. However, once you are familiar with identifying this plant, you can try one and see what you think!

HABITAT

Kwiɫayus occurs in dry open woods and rocky slopes, mostly on the west side of the Cascades from southern BC to central California. It is also found in areas of northern Idaho.

BOTANICAL DESCRIPTION

Kwiɫayus is a shrub that grows between 3–10 feet (1–3 m) tall with reddish-brown bark and crinkled five-lobed leaves that are 0.8–2.5 inches (2–6 cm) across with pale hairy undersides. The pink to deep-red flowers appear in early spring in clusters of ten to twenty. Berries are bluish-black with little sticky hairs and a whitish, waxy surface cast or "bloom."

SUSTAINABLE HARVEST AND TIMING

The blooms of kwiɫayus are ready for harvest in early April. Because you are harvesting a flower that other life rely on, be sure to spread your harvest out and only take what you can use. Remember, only harvest from areas where the shrub is abundant. Berries ripen in June and July, but they are not highly regarded as a food.

PLANT GIFTS

Much of the gift of this plant is purely in its presence on the land. The beauty of the blooms stands out. The flowers can be harvested for a variety of uses. One lovely and simple preparation is to place freshly harvested flowers into a glass container of filtered water, let the water infuse in the sun, and then drink the infusion to enjoy the delicate flavor. The bark has been utilized to make a tea and can also be used as an eyewash for sore eyes.

Kwiɫayus-Infused Honey
1 cup (240 ml)

1 cup (25 g) kwiɫayus blossoms
1 cup (240 ml) honey

1   Pour water in the bottom pot of a double boiler, being careful not to have the water touching the bottom of the top pot. Place the blossoms and honey in the top pot. Simmer the honey on low to medium heat, checking throughout that the water in the bottom pot has not evaporated.

2   Let the mixture infuse for 2 hours. While still warm, pour the honey through a strainer (sieve off the blossoms and then compost the discarded blossoms) into a clean mason jar.

You can also do a cold infusion by placing the same amounts of honey and blossoms as you would for the hot infusion into a mason jar and letting the mixture sit for 6 weeks. Be sure to stir the blossoms with this method so the honey can fully saturate all the blossoms. Strain out the blossoms after the 6 weeks.

T'áḵa7ay

t-ahk-ah

SALAL

Gaultheria shallon

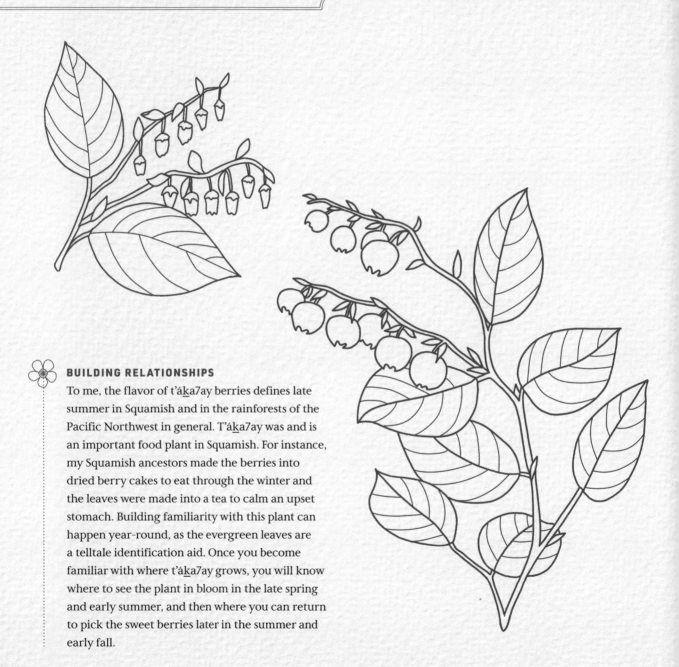

🌸 BUILDING RELATIONSHIPS

To me, the flavor of t'áḵa7ay berries defines late summer in Squamish and in the rainforests of the Pacific Northwest in general. T'áḵa7ay was and is an important food plant in Squamish. For instance, my Squamish ancestors made the berries into dried berry cakes to eat through the winter and the leaves were made into a tea to calm an upset stomach. Building familiarity with this plant can happen year-round, as the evergreen leaves are a telltale identification aid. Once you become familiar with where t'áḵa7ay grows, you will know where to see the plant in bloom in the late spring and early summer, and then where you can return to pick the sweet berries later in the summer and early fall.

HABITAT

T'ák̲a7ay grows in dry to wet forests as well as in bogs and on coastal bluffs, headlands, and shorelines in low to mid elevations. It is common and often abundant along the Pacific coast from southeast Alaska to western BC, Washington, Oregon, and Southern California.

BOTANICAL DESCRIPTION

T'ák̲a7ay is an evergreen shrub that reaches up to 0.98–10 feet (0.3–3 m) in height and can grow erect, sprawling, or partially creeping with stiff crooked stems and sticky twigs. It keeps its beautiful broad, oval-shaped, lustrous green leaves through the winter. It can grow rapidly, with masses of white or pink bell-shaped flowers from May–June and plentiful dark-purple edible berries in the fall.

SUSTAINABLE HARVEST AND TIMING

T'ák̲a7ay grows many berries on a single branch, making them relatively easy to harvest, yet care must be taken to not take too many berries from one area. Bears and other non-human life rely on this berry for food as well, so spreading out your harvest is important. Berries ripen in late August to September. The berries are quite soft, so you still need to pick gently so as not to crush them.

PLANT GIFTS

The berries form in late summer and were traditionally mashed and made into cakes to store for use through the winter. They are sweet and delicious and are very high in antioxidants. The branches make the best whisk for making soapberry whip (see page 123)! The deep purple berries are rich in antioxidants and are sweet but not too juicy, making them perfect for preserving in fruit leather or mixing into jams. Blend the t'ák̲a7ay berries with thimbleberry (see page 127) for a decadent fruit leather.

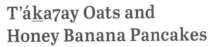

T'ák̲a7ay Oats and Honey Banana Pancakes

10–12 pancakes

1 cup (90 g) rolled oats
2 bananas
3 eggs
2 teaspoons honey
½ teaspoon ground cinnamon
¼ teaspoon baking powder
Butter or coconut oil
1 cup (148 g) fresh t'ák̲a7ay berries, plus more for serving
Maple syrup, for serving

1. In a food processor or blender, pulverize the oats until they become a coarse flour.

2. Add the bananas, eggs, honey, cinnamon, and baking powder to the oat flour and mix the ingredients together in the food processor or blender until a batter is formed. Scrape down the sides of the food processor or blender with a spatula as needed.

3. Warm a medium frying pan over medium heat. Place a little butter or coconut oil in the pan and allow it to melt and warm up briefly.

4. Pour ¼ cup (60 ml) of the pancake batter into the pan. Then spread a tablespoon of t'ák̲a7ay berries evenly on top of the pancake batter and let it fry for 2 minutes with the pan covered.

5. Flip the pancake and fry it covered for another minute.

6. Repeat until all your batter and berries are used up.

7. Serve with some maple syrup and more t'ák̲a7ay berries over the top.

Yetwánaý

yet-wan-eye

SALMONBERRY

Rubus spectabilis

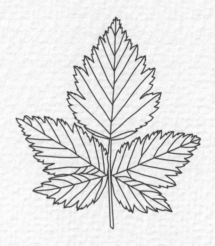

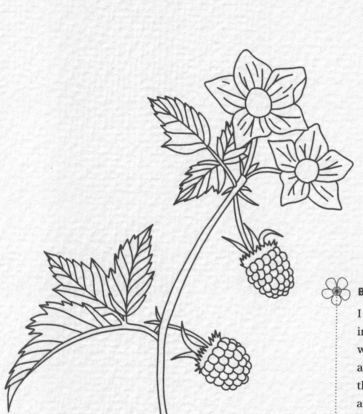

BUILDING RELATIONSHIPS

I recall walking with my dad through the forest in spring when he spotted a saskay (the Squamish word for salmonberry shoot); he leaned down and picked one that was just right. He told me that they should be about as bendable as licorice and slightly red in color. Then he showed me how to peel the thin outer skin from the juicy shoot. The fresh, crisp, green flavor carried notes of the berry. I thought how incredible it must have been for my ancestors to have come through a long winter and to have their first taste of saskays in the spring.

HABITAT

Yetwánaý grows in the dappled shade of moist to wet forests and swamps, along streambanks and shores, and in thickets and clearings, at low to mid elevations from the southern coast of Alaska to Northern California and mostly west of the Pacific coast to the Cascade Mountains.

BOTANICAL DESCRIPTION

Yetwánaý is a thicket-forming, erect to arching shrub, usually 3–10 feet (1–3 m) tall. It has papery reddish-brown bark with scattered prickles on the stem and branches. Leaves have three leaflets that are dark green and sharply toothed. Flowers are large, about 1.2 inches (3 cm) across, and pink to red or magenta. Berries range in color from yellow, to orange, to reddish.

SUSTAINABLE HARVEST AND TIMING

The saskays come up in late March/early April and bloom in April–May. The fruit ripens in May–July. The flowers can be harvested sparingly for use as garnish on desserts or salads—but again, when harvesting flowers, you are taking part of the plant away that is needed for the pollination that enables fruit to develop. Once the berries appear, spread out your harvest across sites with ample bushes, as these berries are food for wildlife as well.

PLANT GIFTS

The gifts of yetwánaý are many. The saskays are a nutritious food rich in minerals and vitamin C and are also a wonderful source of fiber. The berries are a favorite early summer snack. They can be eaten fresh, integrated into recipes such as smoothies and berry compotes, or frozen for use later in the year. There is a teaching in Squamish and from other Indigenous communities about the relationship between yetwánaý and the Swainson's thrush or salmonberry bird. The belief is that the song of this bird ripens the salmonberries and signals when they are ready for harvest.

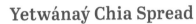

Yetwánaý Chia Spread

1½ cups (510 g)

¼ cup (41 g) chia seeds
1 cup (240 ml) water
¼ cup (52 g) cane sugar
1 cup (125 g) fresh yetwánaý

1 Soak the chia seeds in water for 1 hour. Stir a few times during the first 5 minutes to ensure all seeds are under the water.

2 Once the chia seeds are gelatinous, place them into a blender with the cane sugar and yetwánaý and blend until all the ingredients are combined.

3 If you prefer a spread with no seeds (yetwánaý can be very seedy), use a cheesecloth to strain out the seeds. It will make the spread a bit runnier but still delicious. You can also add 2 more tablespoons of chia seeds to the spread once you have strained it to thicken it up if you want. To do so, stir in the extra chia seeds and let sit for an hour before using.

4 Serve with your favorite morning toast or afternoon crackers. Or, store the spread for up to 2 weeks in an airtight container in your refrigerator.

Nástaḿaý

n-aw-stem-eye

SASKATOON BERRY

Amelanchier alnifolia

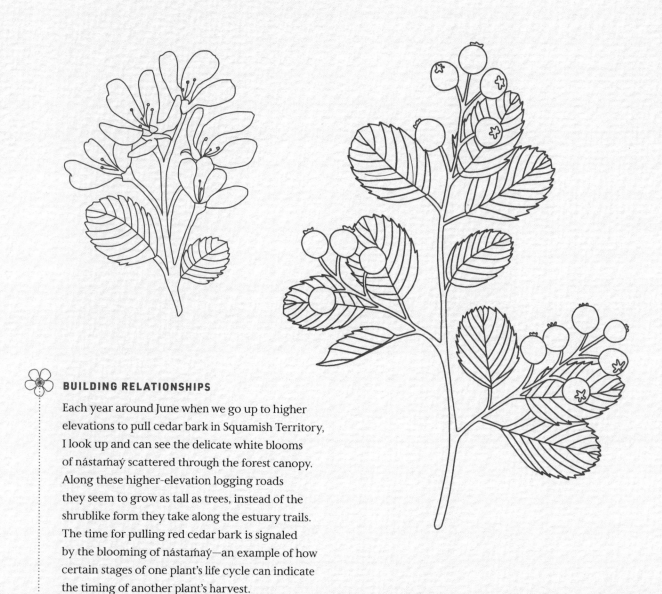

BUILDING RELATIONSHIPS

Each year around June when we go up to higher
elevations to pull cedar bark in Squamish Territory,
I look up and can see the delicate white blooms
of nástaḿaý scattered through the forest canopy.
Along these higher-elevation logging roads
they seem to grow as tall as trees, instead of the
shrublike form they take along the estuary trails.
The time for pulling red cedar bark is signaled
by the blooming of nástaḿaý—an example of how
certain stages of one plant's life cycle can indicate
the timing of another plant's harvest.

HABITAT

Nástaḿaý grows in a variety of dry to moist, well-drained habitats from rocky shorelines, stream banks, and open forests to grasslands and rocky slopes at low to mid elevations. It grows from Alaska to California in the west and eastward to Quebec and in the United States to western Colorado, northern Nebraska, and Iowa.

BOTANICAL DESCRIPTION

Nástaḿaý is a shrub, or rarely a small tree, that grows on average 3–20 feet (1–6 m) tall, and sometimes up to 33 feet (10 m). The slender stems and twigs have smooth, reddish-brown to greyish bark. The leaf margins are saw-toothed, more deeply so along the top half of the leaf edge. This feature is helpful in identifying nástaḿaý, especially when it isn't in flower or fruit. The showy flowers are white and starlike with narrow petals. The ripe fruits are small and berrylike (technically mini apples), and are reddish purple to nearly black in color.

SUSTAINABLE HARVEST AND TIMING

When harvesting the berries, be sure to spread out your harvest to leave enough berries on the tree for other life that rely on them. Nástaḿaý is an excellent candidate for planting in your garden.

PLANT GIFTS

The berries can be picked and eaten fresh off the branch or dried and utilized later. Not all berries can dry well, but nástaḿaý is not a particularly juicy berry, so it pairs well with thimbleberry and salal in wildberry fruit leathers!

Seedy Nástaḿaý Granola Bread

12–14 pieces

3 tablespoons coconut oil
1½ cup (360 ml) hot water
¼ cup (60 ml) maple syrup
½ cup (70 g) pumpkin seeds
1 cup (140 g) almonds
1 cup (140 g) sunflower seeds
1½ cups (135 g) rolled oats
½ teaspoon sea salt
½ cup (80 g) hemp seed hearts
1 cup (140 g) raisins
½ cup (74 g) nástaḿaý (or other berries of your choice)

1 Preheat the oven to 350°F (175°C).

2 In a large bowl, add the coconut oil, hot water, and maple syrup. Mix using a spatula.

3 Add all the remaining ingredients to the bowl except the nástaḿaý and mix until well combined.

4 Place the mixture in a food processor and gently blend until everything is incorporated but not to the point it becomes a smooth batter. You want the mixture to be a bit chunky.

5 Fold in the nástaḿaý.

6 Place the bread mixture on parchment paper in a medium baking dish. Press it down evenly with a fork until about 1 inch (2.5 cm) thick.

7 Bake in the oven for 30 minutes.

8 If you want the bread to be crunchier, flip the bread to the other side and bake for another 20 minutes.

9 Once done, let cool for 30 minutes.

10 Cut the bread into your desired serving size. You can freeze pieces for up to 3 months, or keep in the refrigerator for up to 7 days.

S̱xwúsum

s-xw-oh-sum

SOAPBERRY

Shepherdia canadensis

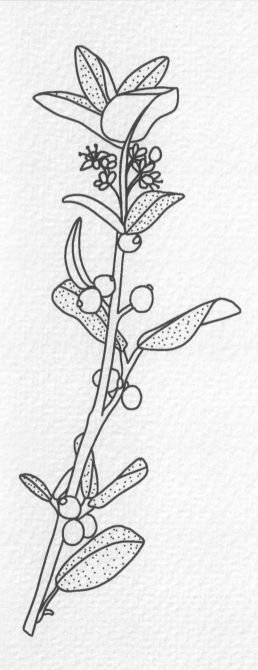

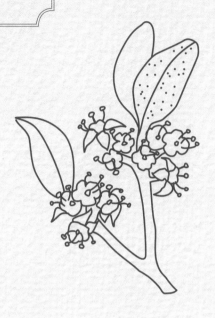

 BUILDING RELATIONSHIPS

S̱xwúsum is a plant that does not commonly grow in the Squamish region, but it has been received in trade with neighboring Indigenous nations, including Líl̓wat in what is now present-day Pemberton, BC. When I lived in northern BC and the Yukon, this plant was everywhere! It was so amazing to see it growing in my front yard. Each year my family would go out and pick the sticky berries and taste some while we picked. The berries are very bitter as they contain a compound called saponin, which also makes them froth up when whipped. I first tasted this berry whip when I was little. The bitter fruits, often mixed with a sweetener like sugar, give this delicacy its unique flavor.

HABITAT

Sx̱wúsum grows in dry to mesic sites including open forests, forest edges, and thickets. It also grows on rocky outcrops and ridges, from the lowlands up into the subalpine. It is common throughout most of BC, but is absent on Haida Gwaii, northern Vancouver Island, and the adjacent north coast. Sx̱wúsum grows north up to Alaska and Yukon, and south down to Washington and Oregon.

BOTANICAL DESCRIPTION

Sx̱wúsum is a deciduous shrub standing 3–10 feet (1–3 m) tall. The branches are covered in small coppery scales. Leaves are opposite and elliptical to narrowly oval and are 0.5–2 inches (1.3–5 cm) long and 0.4–1.1 inches (1–3 cm) wide. They are greenish with a whitish felt on the upper surface and coppery scales beneath. The flowers are tiny, yellowish, and without petals. The fruit are bright red berries that are soapy when touched and grow only on the female plants.

SUSTAINABLE HARVEST AND TIMING

The berries ripen in the summer months. The exact timing may vary across geographic range. When the berries are red and begin to soften, they are ready for harvest. Bears and birds love these berries, so spread out your harvest with their access to this food in mind. The berries can be soft; you can gently shake the branches or comb them with your fingers over a basket or sheet to catch them as they fall.

PLANT GIFTS

Sx̱wúsum carries many gifts. The berries or juice can be consumed to calm an upset stomach, have been used to treat high blood pressure, and are rich in vitamin C. The juice can also be applied topically to treat acne or boils. As a food, the bitter berries are made into a soapberry whip (sometimes called soopalalie) that is enjoyed as a dessert by many Indigenous communities.

Sx̱wúsum Whip

about 2 quarts (320 g)

¼ cup (40 g) fresh or frozen sx̱wúsum (defrosted if frozen)
2 tablespoons water, plus more if needed
2 tablespoons sugar, plus more if needed (optional)
½ banana, sliced (optional)

1   In a large bowl, press the sx̱wúsum through a fine-mesh sieve. (This is optional, but results in a smoother consistency.)

2   Add the water to the pressed sx̱wúsum. Use an electric mixer to beat the berries and water. After a few minutes, soft meringue-like peaks should begin to form. This may take longer than you think!

3   If you are using sugar, add it after stiff peaks have formed. Start with 2 tablespoons and adjust to taste. For a version without refined sugar, try adding sliced banana while the electric mixer is still running. Blend until the banana is completely incorporated, and the soapberry mix has formed stiff peaks.

   Other berries can be used to sweeten the whip as well: try saskatoon, blueberries, or salal berries!

Séliýaý

s-elle-ee-eye

TALL OREGON GRAPE

Mahonia aquifolium

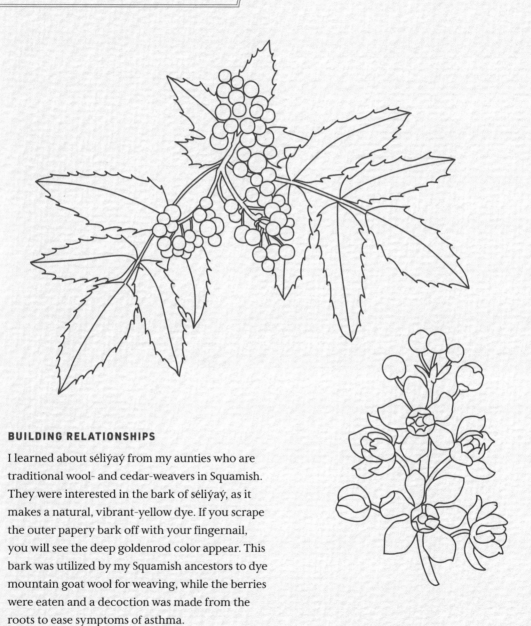

BUILDING RELATIONSHIPS

I learned about séliýaý from my aunties who are traditional wool- and cedar-weavers in Squamish. They were interested in the bark of séliýaý, as it makes a natural, vibrant-yellow dye. If you scrape the outer papery bark off with your fingernail, you will see the deep goldenrod color appear. This bark was utilized by my Squamish ancestors to dye mountain goat wool for weaving, while the berries were eaten and a decoction was made from the roots to ease symptoms of asthma.

HABITAT

Séliẏaẏ grows in open, usually coniferous forests and forest edges, and on rock outcrops and rocky slopes at low to mid elevations. It is found along the Pacific coast from southern BC to Northern California and inland across BC, Washington, and northern Idaho to the Rockies.

BOTANICAL DESCRIPTION

Séliẏaẏ is an evergreen shrub that grows 6–8 feet (2–2.4 m) tall, spreading by underground stems and aboveground runners to form stands about 5 feet (1.5 m) wide. The stems and branches have yellow inner bark and wood. Séliẏaẏ has compound leaves; each leaf has five to nine leathery leaflets with one central vein per leaflet. The shiny, evergreen leaflets have spiny-toothed margins and are holly-like in appearance. Brilliant yellow flowers are borne in terminal clusters, followed by dark blue, large-seeded, grapelike berries about 0.4 inch (1 cm) across and with a silvery bloom on the surface.

SUSTAINABLE HARVEST AND TIMING

When harvesting the berries, it is easy to take the entire bunch from the plant, but be sure to leave some on each plant for other life that rely on them. Bring clippers so you can easily take part of the bunch of berries and leave some behind. If harvesting the bark, I look to clip straight branches, and am careful to take only one or two from a single plant. Please conduct more research on how to sustainably harvest the root of séliẏaẏ, as doing so takes much care and knowledge.

PLANT GIFTS

Séliẏaẏ contains the compound berberine, which is a liver stimulant and is strongly antimicrobial. If you do not carry the knowledge and expertise to ingest this plant as a medicine, seek guidance from an expert herbalist first. The berries are tart and rich in antioxidants.

Séliẏaẏ Jelly

approximately 2 cups (640 g)

6 cups (900 g) séliẏaẏ berries, cleaned and rinsed
2 cups (480 ml) water
½ pouch (1 to 1½ ounces, or 30 to 45 ml) liquid pectin
½ lemon, juiced (⅛ cup, or 30 ml)
3 cups (600 g) sugar

1   In a large pot, add the berries and water.

2   Bring the water to a boil, then turn down the heat and simmer for 15 minutes. Use a large spoon to crush the berries against the side of the pot to release the juice.

3   Strain the berries through a fine-mesh sieve lined with cheesecloth into a different large pot to remove any seeds.

4   Measure your strained juice/pulp. You should have about 3 cups (720 ml); if you have less, top up with water.

5   Place the pot on the stovetop. Add the liquid pectin and lemon juice. Stir the mixture well and heat on high, stirring consistently, so that the mixture can reduce.

6   Once the mixture is boiling, quickly add the sugar. Return to a rolling boil and boil for exactly 1 minute. Remove the pot from the burner.

7   Place the jelly in clean, hot canning jars. Wipe the tops of the jars to remove any spillage and cover with the lids.

8   Seal the lids on the jars in a hot-water bath for 10 minutes. If any lids do not seal, refrigerate and use within 3 weeks.

T'ák̲w'emaý

t-aw-kw-em-eye
THIMBLEBERRY
Rubus parviflorus

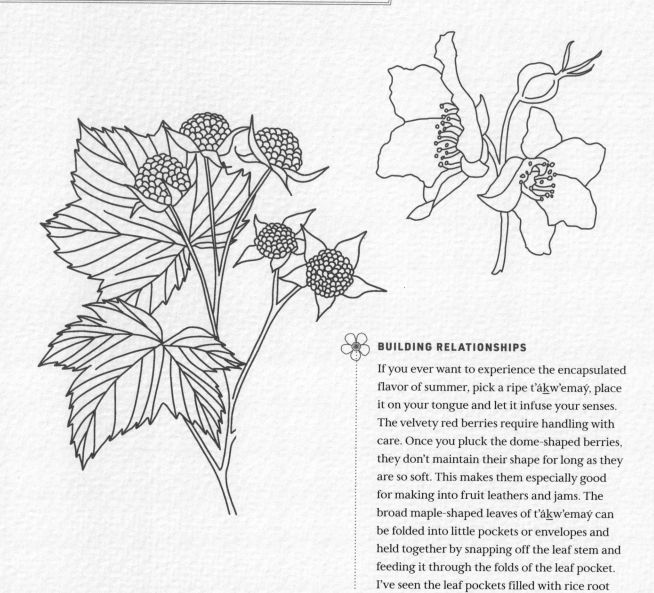

BUILDING RELATIONSHIPS

If you ever want to experience the encapsulated flavor of summer, pick a ripe t'ák̲w'emaý, place it on your tongue and let it infuse your senses. The velvety red berries require handling with care. Once you pluck the dome-shaped berries, they don't maintain their shape for long as they are so soft. This makes them especially good for making into fruit leathers and jams. The broad maple-shaped leaves of t'ák̲w'emaý can be folded into little pockets or envelopes and held together by snapping off the leaf stem and feeding it through the folds of the leaf pocket. I've seen the leaf pockets filled with rice root bulblets to keep them together during the cooking process. The dried leaves have been utilized as a poultice to treat burns and other skin ailments. My Squamish ancestors had a village site called t'ek̲w't'ák̲w'umay, or "place of lots of thimbleberries."

HABITAT

T'ák̲w'emaý grows in moist to mesic open woods, edges, thickets, roadsides, streambanks, clearings, and along shorelines from southeast Alaska to northern Mexico. Eastward, it can be found throughout the Rocky Mountain states and provinces to New Mexico, as well as through South Dakota to the Great Lakes region.

BOTANICAL DESCRIPTION

T'ák̲w'emaý is a medium to tall shrub growing up to 3–8 feet (1–2.5 m) that usually forms dense thickets. The stems are smooth in young plants and are gray and flaky in older plants. The leaves are large, 4–8 inches (10–20 cm) across, maple-like in shape, long-stemmed, and fuzzy on both surfaces. The large, white flowers (about 1.5 inches, or 4 cm) grow in groups of three to seven in a terminal cluster. The raspberry-like fruit is a cluster of small, red, hairy drupelets in the shape of a domed cap.

SUSTAINABLE HARVEST AND TIMING

The flowers bloom in May–June and the fruit ripens in July–September. Be mindful of the other life that rely on the berries and spread out your harvest. The nature of these berries demands careful work, as they are very soft and it takes a long time to harvest them, but the flavor is worth the effort!

PLANT GIFTS

From the spring shoots to the flowers and berries, t'ák̲w'emaý has many gifts to offer. The spring shoots are rich in minerals and vitamin C and can be nibbled right off the plant in the early spring when they are still tender. The berries are rich in vitamin C and antioxidants that are beneficial to your health. And that flavor! The berries taste quintessentially like summer to me.

T'ák̲w'emaý Fruit Leather
14 × 14 inches (35 × 35 cm) fruit sheets

4 cups (560 g) t'ák̲w'emaý (you can mix with other berries like salal and blueberries)
¼ cup (60 ml) water

There are three ways to prepare fruit leather: dehydrate using a dehydrator appliance, oven-dry, and sun-dry.

1   For each of the options, you will first need to blend the t'ák̲w'emaý and water in a blender until the mixture becomes liquid.

2   Once this is done, you can follow the dehydration instructions that fit your desired method (see page 47).

3   For each method, you will pour the blended berries onto the appropriate sheet and spread the mixture evenly and thinly, about 2 inches (5 cm) thick, using a spatula.

4   With any of the methods above, you can store leftover fruit leather in an airtight container in your cupboard for up to 1 month.

Sḵw'elṁxw

sk-wel-m-ooh
TRAILING BLACKBERRY
Rubus ursinus

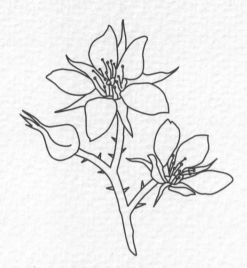

BUILDING RELATIONSHIPS

Sḵw'elṁxw is one of the first plants I was taught about for making tea. The flavor of the leaf carries the sweetness of berries when steeped. One of the first memories I have of trailing blackberry was being tripped by its long and creeping vinelike stems; these create groundcover in parts of the coastal temperate rainforests in the Pacific Northwest and can wrap around your ankle. The delicate white blooms cast a lovely, low canopy over the ground when they are in bloom, and the tiny but flavorful berries are a treat when they ripen. The berries were an important winter food for my Squamish ancestors. They were dried into cakes and the leaves were part of an eye wash medicine.

128

HABITAT

Sḵw'elḿxw grows in dry to moist thickets and in clearings, recent forest fire sites, and areas of cleared forest due to logging, as well as open forests from low to mid elevations. It is common in southwestern BC to Northern California and inland to Idaho.

BOTANICAL DESCRIPTION

Sḵw'elḿxw is a trailing shrub that grows to 7–16 feet (2–5 m) or more long. The stems are 0.07–0.4 inch (2–10 mm) in diameter and grow sprawling and trailing along the ground. Leaves are dark green and comprised of three leaflets with toothed margins. The flowering canes stand upright and are 4–12 inches (10–30 cm) tall and the white to pinkish flowers are approximately 1.5 inches (4 cm) across. The small berries are red at first, but then turn black when ripe. They are egg-shaped and about 0.6 inch (1.5 cm) long.

SUSTAINABLE HARVEST AND TIMING

The delicious berries of sḵw'elḿxw are ripe in July, and though they are tiny, they are flavorful! As with other berries, consider the other life that rely on the berries and do not take too much from one area. Picking these berries is a labor of love. I have mostly just stopped and eaten some of these berries trailside, but if you have the time and self-control to harvest enough for a recipe then you are in for a treat!

PLANT GIFTS

The leaves can be used to make a tea that is flavorful and rich in antioxidants and can help boost immunity. The berries are not only tasty but are also packed full of vitamin C, antioxidants, and fiber.

Sḵw'elḿxw Crumble

6–8 servings

4 cups (576 g) ripe sḵw'elḿxw (you can substitute with any blend of fresh, ripe berries), rinsed
1 cup (207 g) cane sugar or brown sugar
1 teaspoon vanilla extract
1 cup (125 g) all-purpose flour
½ teaspoon salt
1 teaspoon ground cinnamon
¼ teaspoon ground nutmeg
1 tablespoon baking powder
8 tablespoons cubed butter, chilled (you can substitute with an equal amount of coconut oil)
Dairy or nondairy vanilla bean ice cream, for serving

1   Preheat the oven to 375°F (190°C).

2   In a large bowl, use a spatula to combine the rinsed sḵw'elḿxw (or substitutes), sugar, and vanilla.

3   In a separate large bowl, whisk together the flour, salt, cinnamon, nutmeg, and baking powder until well combined. Stir in the butter.

4   Grease or line a 9 × 13-inch (23 x 33-cm) baking pan with parchment paper so that the cobbler will not stick. Then pour in your berry mixture and spread evenly in the pan. Pour the spice topping over the berry mixture.

5   Bake at 375°F (190°C) for 40–45 minutes, or until the topping is golden brown. Serve with vanilla bean ice cream. Enjoy!

Kál̲kay

call-k-eye

WILD ROSE

*Rosa nutkana, R. pisocarpa,
R. gymnocarpa*

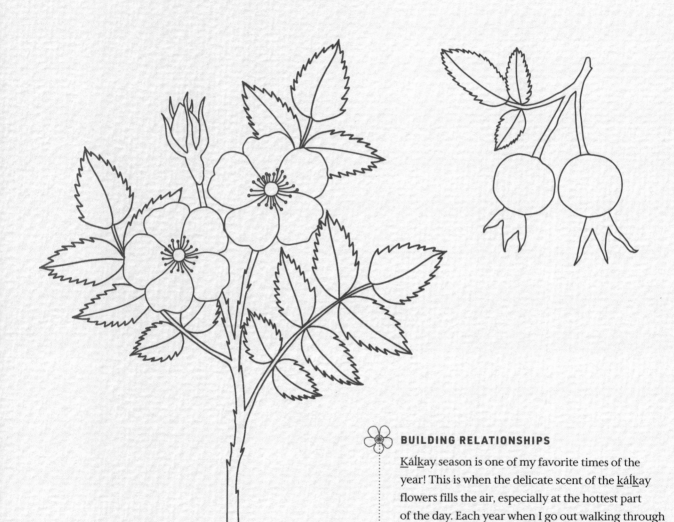

🌼 BUILDING RELATIONSHIPS

Kál̲kay season is one of my favorite times of the year! This is when the delicate scent of the kál̲kay flowers fills the air, especially at the hottest part of the day. Each year when I go out walking through the estuary with my children, it has become a tradition to stop and pick a single kál̲kay petal and place it on our tongues. We close our eyes and let the delicate scent and flavor infuse our senses.

HABITAT

Káḻkay generally grows in open areas, forest and trail edges, thickets, shorelines, and light wooded areas in dry to moist sites at low to mid elevations from Alaska to California, and inland to the Rockies, depending on the species. There are over twenty wild rose species in North America that can be utilized in similar ways; you can do some additional research to determine what species grows in your region. The Sḵwxwú7mesh name for rose covers *Rosa nutkana, R. pisocarpa,* and *R. gymnocarpa.*

BOTANICAL DESCRIPTION

Káḻkay is a shrub that grows between 5–10 feet (1.5–3 m) tall, depending on the species. The shrubs have fairly large compound leaves, meaning they consist of five, seven, or nine smaller, toothed leaflets that are opposite from each other along a central stem. The stems are usually reddish and covered in prickles. In the late spring and early summer, they set rosebuds and then bloom into five-petaled, pale pink to deep rose flowers that, in some species, grow up to 1.1–2.7 inches (3–7 cm) across. Shiny red rosehips develop in late August and can stay on the shrub through the winter if they are not all eaten by birds and other wildlife.

SUSTAINABLE HARVEST AND TIMING

The leaves and stems can be harvested in early spring, and the flowers in the summer. The bright red fruit of the rose can be harvested in the fall after the first frost for enhanced sweetness. This plant is excellent for wildlife habitat enhancement and can be planted in landscaping in various regions. The fragrant flowers bloom from May to July. This is also the time for harvesting the petals, but it is important to leave two to three petals on each flower so pollinators can still land on them. This allows the flowers to develop into the fruit káḻk (rosehips), which are an important food to many bird and mammal species (including humans).

PLANT GIFTS

You can eat most parts of the rose plant. The petals can be eaten fresh and added to salads or made into jams or jellies. The rosehips are very high in vitamin C and can be used to make fruit leathers, syrup, jams, and jellies, but care needs to be taken to clean out the hairy seeds before ingesting the hips, as they are irritating to the digestive tract. The leaves are astringent, and the fruit is antimicrobial and diuretic. Rose petals can be made into a tea and enjoyed hot or cold, or the tea can also be used as an eyewash for irritated eyes.

Good Morning Káḻkay-Petal Protein Shake

2 servings

1 (14-ounce, or 400-ml) can coconut milk
2 cups (480 ml) water
1 cup (125 g) raspberries, frozen or fresh
1 banana, frozen or fresh
1½ tablespoons dried káḻkay petals
¼ cup (40 g) hemp seed hearts
2 tablespoons maple syrup
1 tablespoon pine pollen (optional)

Place all the ingredients into a blender and blend until smooth. Enjoy!

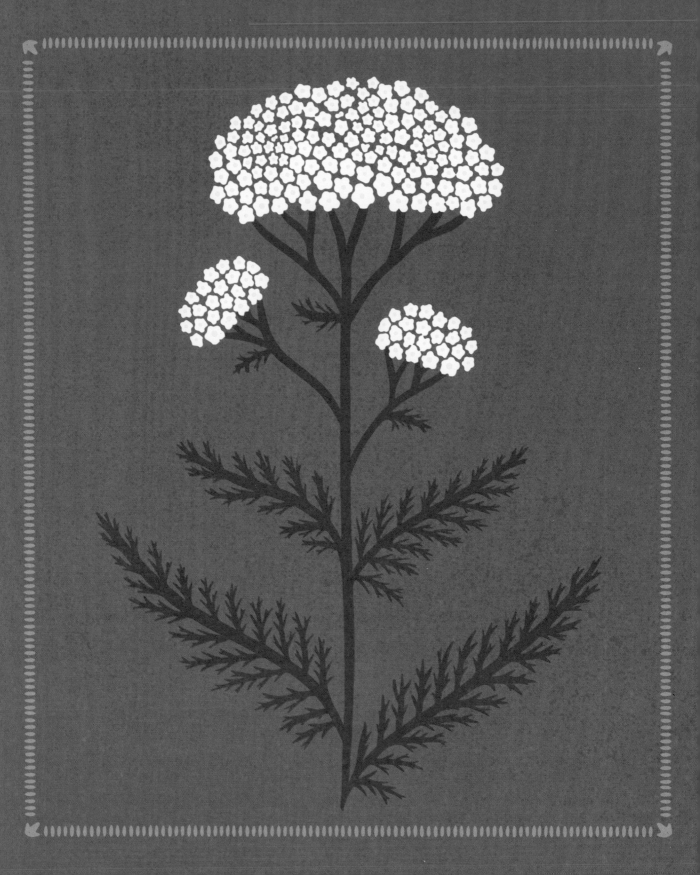

FLOWERING HERBS

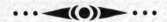

K'exmín

k-uh-x-main

BARE-STEM DESERT PARSLEY OR BISCUITROOT

Lomatium nudicaule

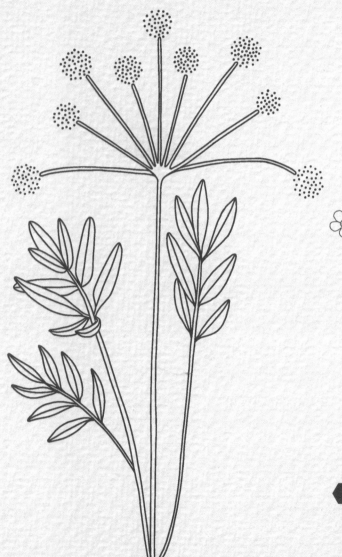

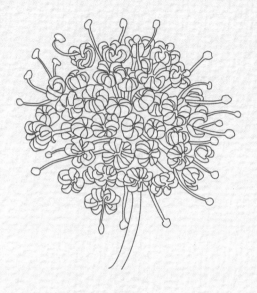

 BUILDING RELATIONSHIPS

K'exmín is a special plant. The seeds are one of the most highly regarded spiritual and physical medicines for many Indigenous communities within its range. The lacy foliage and yellow flowers have such a beauty to them. I remember the first time I saw k'exmín growing; it was in a camas meadow. Camas meadows are traditionally managed ecosystems that have relied historically on seasonal burning to keep the meadows open and productive. I glimpsed the delicate yellow flowers and lacy foliage, and felt so happy to see the plant that yields the treasured k'exmín seeds.

! **WARNING:** *Develop your confidence with identifying this plant as there are other, inedible plant seeds that may look similar to the untrained eye.*

HABITAT

This species thrives in a wide range of habitats, from dry, open, rocky or grassy slopes, and dunes, to seasonally moist meadows and open forests from low to mid elevations. K'exmín often grows in traditionally managed camas meadow ecosystems and its presence in these meadows is concentrated on Vancouver Island, Gulf and San Juan Islands, Puget Sound, and Willamette Valley. The growing range of k'exmín generally extends from southern BC to California, east to southwestern Alberta, and south to the Great Basin regions in Oregon, Nevada, and Utah.

BOTANICAL DESCRIPTION

K'exmín is a striking native carrot-family species that grows to 8–35 inches (20–89 cm) tall, with yellow globe-shaped flowers on long petioles. The bluish-green foliage grows mostly toward the base of the plant, and the leaves are oblong. The stems are hairless. The seeds are oblong, 0.3–0.6 inch (8–15 mm) long, and distinctly striped.

SUSTAINABLE HARVEST AND TIMING

As mentioned, k'exmín is a culturally important plant food and medicine that is difficult to find and harvest due to habitat loss. Please do not wild harvest this plant. I encourage you to research the cultural importance of the plant and grow it in your own garden. If you live in an area where the plant holds cultural importance, you can offer to grow extra for the local Indigenous community. Leaves can be harvested in the spring, and seeds are ready in the late summer/fall.

PLANT GIFTS

K'exmín leaves are celery-flavored, rich in vitamin C, and can be eaten fresh or used to season cooking. The seeds have a multitude of uses, including treating sore throats, coughs, and headaches, as well as being burned as an incense for cleansing spaces. This plant is connected to many ceremonial and spiritual practices for Indigenous Peoples.

Throat-Soothing Tea
1 serving

1 cup (240 ml) boiling water
3–5 k'exmín seeds, dried
½ tablespoon licorice fern (see page 166), dried and cut into pieces

1   Pour the boiling water over the ingredients, either loose in a cup or contained in a tea ball.

2   Let the ingredients steep for 15–20 minutes. Strain out or reserve the seeds and licorice fern rhizome for composting, then enjoy.

Slhí7lhaẃiń tl'a wex̱és

s-th-eh-th-ow-wayn tl'a wa-x-es
BROAD-LEAVED PLANTAIN
Plantago spp.

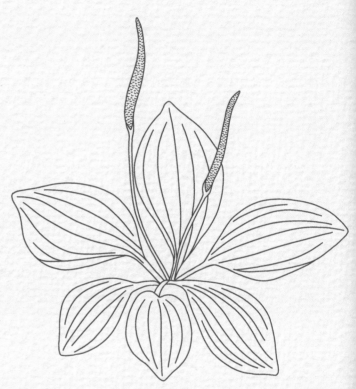

BUILDING RELATIONSHIPS

When I first started teaching in Squamish with youth and community members, one of the first plants people started asking me about was a plant called "frog leaf." It took me a while to figure out they were referring to plantain (*Plantago*) species. The Squamish name, slhí7lhaẃiń tl'a wex̱és, translates to "little bed of the frog." This plant was introduced from Europe and is often considered a weed, but it has such an array of nutritional and topical uses!

HABITAT

The different *Plantago* species grow in a range of habitats and geographic locations. Two of the common plantain species in this region are *P. macrocarpa* and *P. lanceolata*. *P. macrocarpa*, commonly called Alaska plantain, is found growing at low elevations in wet sites such as upper tidal marshes, moist beaches, bogs, and shorelines from Alaska down the coast to Washington. *P. lanceolata*, or English plantain, is commonly found growing along roadsides, in fields and lawns, and disturbed sites and is most concentrated in southwestern BC into Washington. Be sure to research the species in your region for more specific information.

BOTANICAL DESCRIPTION

Slhí7lhaẃiń tl'a wex̱és is a leafy green plant that grows anywhere from 2–6 inches (5–15 cm) tall, depending on the species. The leaves are basal and range from lance-shaped to broad and oval. The flowers grow on spikes and are tiny and green to brown in color. The leaves tend to have strong veins that run parallel.

SUSTAINABLE HARVEST AND TIMING

Generally, slhí7lhaẃiń tl'a wex̱és is plentiful depending on what species you are harvesting. You may decide to harvest more sparingly if the stand of plants is very small and more specialized, like *P. maritima* (sea plantain). This plant will also thrive in a garden box. Slhí7lhaẃiń tl'a wex̱és can be harvested from May through to September but they will be the most tender for eating earlier in the year.

PLANT GIFTS

Slhí7lhaẃiń tl'a wex̱és is edible and can be utilized topically. The leaves are very calming and soothing to the skin when applied as a poultice or ointment. The simplest way to apply the leaves is to chew or grind them up and place them directly on minor cuts, scrapes, or bug bites. The leaves of *P. lanceolata* and *P. macrocarpa* can be made into delicious and nutritional chips by cleaning, seasoning, and roasting them in the oven. Or turn them into a mineral-rich green juice!

Slhí7lhaẃiń tl'a wex̱és Lip Balm

3 ounces (85 g)

NOTE: *You will need three 1-ounce (28-g) metal tins, or fifteen–twenty 0.2-ounce (5-g) lip balm tubes. You may also want a lip balm tray and scraper.*

2 tablespoons dried slhí7lhaẃiń tl'a wex̱és leaves
2 tablespoons coconut oil
1 tablespoon cocoa butter
1 tablespoon sweet almond oil
2 tablespoons beeswax
¼ teaspoon (approximately 25 drops) peppermint
  essential oil

1   Place the slhí7lhaẃiń tl'a wex̱és leaves in a square of cheesecloth and tie the cloth securely with twine.

2   In a double boiler, pour water in the bottom pot, being careful not to have the water touching the bottom of the top pot. Add the coconut oil, cocoa butter, sweet almond oil, and the bundle of slhí7lhaẃiń tl'a wex̱és leaves to the top pot.

3   Warm the mixture over medium heat for 1 hour. Be sure to add water to the bottom pot so it does not evaporate completely.

4   After 1 hour, carefully remove the slhí7lhaẃiń tl'a wex̱és-leaf bundle and squeeze out any excess oil using tongs. Compost the slhí7lhaẃiń tl'a wex̱és leaves.

5   If there are leaf particles in the oil, you may want to strain them through a fine-mesh sieve to remove them. Place the strained oil back into the double boiler.

6   Add the beeswax and melt it over medium heat in the top of the double boiler.

7   Once the ingredients are all melted, turn off the heat and let the oil mixture cool to 130–140°F (54–60°C). Add the essential oil. Waiting until the oils have cooled ensures the essential oil will not evaporate when added.

8   Pour the lip balm mixture carefully into chosen lip balm containers. For lip balm tubes you can order special trays to hold the tubes while you fill them. Look at your local craft or DIY supply store for these and for lip balm scrapers to remove the excess lip balm from the tops of the tubes before putting on the lids.

Spánanexw

sp-awn-awn-exw

CAMAS

Camassia leichtlinii (great camas),
C. quamash (common camas)

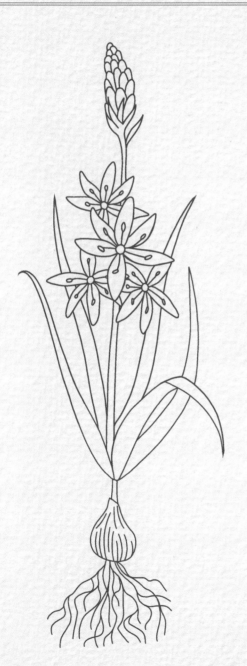

BUILDING RELATIONSHIPS

Spánanexw is a special plant: a nutritious, delicious root vegetable that has been cultivated in specialized meadow ecosystems that are managed through seasonal burning, weeding, and selective harvesting of key root vegetables. These meadows, sometimes referred to as camas or Garry oak meadow ecosystems, are one of the clearest examples of intensive Indigenous plant management. Spánanexw bulbs were traded to neighboring Indigenous communities as a highly valued food. Seeing a meadow of spánanexw in bloom in the early spring is a beautiful sight to behold. There are efforts in some Indigenous communities to bring back the seasonal burning to renew and maintain the very small amount of spánanexw habitat that remains.

HABITAT

Spánanexw grows in the springtime in mesic to moist meadows, grasslands, and oak woodland at low to mid elevations. It is concentrated on southern Vancouver Island, the Gulf Islands, and San Juan Islands in the Salish Sea, and south through Puget Sound and Willamette Valley to California, extending to the Rockies.

BOTANICAL DESCRIPTION

Spánanexw is a perennial herb from a white bulb that is 0.8–1.6 inches (2–4 cm) long. The smooth, flowering stems grow between 8–39 inches (20–100 cm) tall. Leaves are basal, clumped, narrow, and grasslike. They can grow up to

6–20 inches (15–50 cm) long and 0.4–0.8 inch (1–2 cm) wide. Oblong, egg-shaped capsules produce many shiny black seeds 0.08–0.15 inch (2–4 mm) long. The pale to deep blue flowers have six petals that, when withered, twist together over the capsules in great camas but not in common camas.

SUSTAINABLE HARVEST AND TIMING

Spánanexw habitat has been highly impacted, and it is not advised to harvest this bulb unless you have Indigenous heritage in a region where this plant grows. However, this plant can be purchased from native plant nurseries and grown in a garden. Spánanexw bulbs are harvested in the summer months; some people suggest waiting until the plant goes to seed. When harvesting the bulbs, it is important to do this with the plant still attached so you can be sure you have the correct bulb.

PLANT GIFTS

Spánanexw is a highly valued food plant. The bulb is highly nutritious and was a rare source of carbohydrates in an Indigenous diet. The bulbs have a starch called inulin. When the bulbs are properly prepared by slow roasting for 24–48 hours, the inulin breaks down to fructose and sweetens and caramelizes the bulbs, making them a delicious delicacy. The bulbs were once traded extensively with Indigenous Peoples in communities where spánanexw didn't grow.

For this plant I will include information on how to plant spánanexw in your garden in lieu of a recipe. Many Indigenous communities engaged in restoration efforts of this culturally important plant food are concerned about overharvesting. Planting spánanexw is a good way to contribute to the solution and not the problem.

Grow Spánanexw

Spánanexw bulbs or seeds purchased from a native plant nursery
Raised bed, garden bed, or large pots or containers

1   In nature, spánanexw grows in meadows and the edges of open woods. In a garden setting, it thrives in full sun to partial shade in well-drained soils that dry out between watering. You can plant spánanexw in containers, raised beds, or the edges of garden beds. This gorgeous purple bloom will flower in May to June and draw pollinators to your garden. I have had success growing spánanexw in smaller pots to raised beds that are around 1.5–2 feet (0.5–0.6 m) deep with soil.

2   If growing from seed, the seeds need 60–90 days of cold-moist stratification (or "winterization") in order to break down the seed coat and trigger springtime seed germination. (If you are unfamiliar with this process, I encourage you to do more research on it.) The freeze-thaw cycle, rain, snow, and general winter conditions contribute to successful spring germination. If the seeds are sown too late, they won't achieve the required cold stratification and will remain dormant until the following spring.

3   Once you have an established bed of spánanexw, you can dig up, separate, and replant them to grow the numbers.

4   Consider sharing the spánanexw bulbs with the local Indigenous community if spánanexw was historically cultivated in the area you live.

Sts'á7<u>k</u>in

s-ts-ah-kane
CATTAIL
Typha latifolia

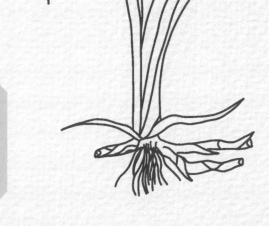

BUILDING RELATIONSHIPS

Sts'á7<u>k</u>in is a prolific plant in the Squamish Estuary and it provides many options as a food source. Each spring I go to the Squamish Estuary and see the new shoots of the sts'á7<u>k</u>in plants popping up. Later in the summer the tall stalks will cover whole large areas of the estuary; their gray-green leaves and brown, cylindrical heads will move with the wind and provide habitat for migratory bird species. One of my favorite sights is to see a red-winged blackbird singing atop a sts'á7<u>k</u>in flower head.

WARNING: *Be careful not to confuse sts'á7<u>k</u>in with poisonous iris species which may be found growing in the same environments. Only harvest sts'á7<u>k</u>in when you are one hundred percent confident of your identification.*

HABITAT

Sts'á7kin grows in very wet habitats such as marshes, lake shores, ponds, wet ditches, and in languid or still waters, at low to mid elevations. It is common in southern BC and infrequent in northeastern BC. Sts'á7kin is widespread in North America. It is found in all states, provinces, and territories except Nunavut, up north to Alaska and the Yukon, and south to California and Mexico.

BOTANICAL DESCRIPTION

Sts'á7kin is a semiaquatic, perennial herb growing from a tough, extensive system of rhizomes. The stems stand straight and grow up to 39–118 inches (100–300 cm) tall and are hard and round in a cross section. Leaves are flat, about 0.31–0.8 inch (8–20 mm) wide, and taper to tips. The tiny flowers are numerous and sit in a cylindrical spike atop the stem. The seeds are dry, long, and hairy, measuring about 0.04 inch (1 mm) long.

SUSTAINABLE HARVEST AND TIMING

Depending on what part of the plant you are harvesting, the timing will vary. For harvesting the spring shoots, you will want to go out before the flower spike grows in order to catch the shoots while they are still tender (this is usually in May in my region). For the pollen, you will want to harvest in June. The rhizomes can be harvested year-round, but are best in the fall and winter after the aboveground part of the plant has started to die back.

PLANT GIFTS

The entire plant is edible, including the pollen, shoots, and roots. As a result, this plant is a productive and reliable food source. The leaves of sts'á7kin have been historically utilized to weave multipurpose mats, a practice which is coming back in some Indigenous communities. The rhizome provided an important source of carbohydrates to my Squamish ancestors. Be careful to know the history of your harvest site, as there are, for example, industrial sites in the Squamish Estuary that still have contaminated soil.

Sts'á7kin Flour

½–1 cup (63–125 g)

10–15 sts'á7kin roots
Cooking oil, for greasing

1 Scrape and clean the roots to remove the thick, spongy outer skin, as well as any dirt.

2 Place the root cores on a lightly greased baking tray.

3 Slowly warm and dry the roots in a 200°F (95°C) oven overnight. Or place on a drying rack for 2 days.

4 Pound the roots with a tool like a kitchen mallet until you have a fine powder, removing any fibers. You may need to run the flour through a fine-mesh sieve to remove fibers.

5 Let the flour sit overnight to dry further.

6 Sift and use as a flour or cornstarch alternative to thicken stew or gravy.

Yúla7

yo-la
COW PARSNIP
Heracleum maximum

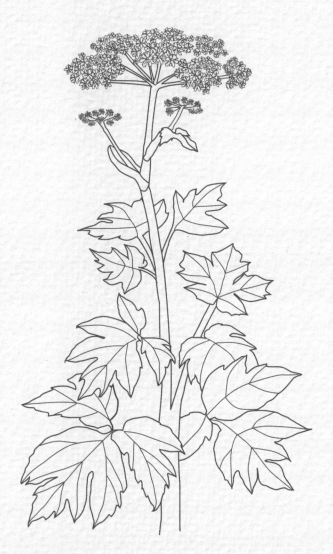

 BUILDING RELATIONSHIPS

Yúla7 is an early spring green that I first learned about while living in northern BC in Tahltan territory. We had a community garden just outside of town along one of the rivers, and yúla7 was one of the first edible spring foods to grow abundantly at the garden site. The bright-green shoots come up in the early spring and signal the start of the wild food growing season. Care needs to be taken when harvesting yúla7 as the sap is phototoxic. That means skin can blister if exposed to sunlight after touching the sap, so be sure to use gloves and clippers when harvesting. There is a Squamish word, "p'elp'áĺaḵi," which refers to a condition where your skin would start to peel after handling yúla7.

 WARNING: *Sharpen your identification of cow parsnip because it looks similar to giant hogweed* (Heracleum mantegazzianum), *which has strongly phototoxic compounds that can cause severe burns to skin. Yúla7 can also be confused with deadly poisonous plants such as poison hemlock* (Conium maculatum) *and water hemlock* (Cicuta douglasii *or* C. maculata). *If you lack the experience to identify this plant with complete confidence, purchase one from a native plant nursery and grow it in your garden instead.*

HABITAT

Yúla7 grows in wet to moist habitats including meadows, open forests, seepage slopes, streambanks, gullies, upper beaches and tidal marshes, avalanche tracks, clearings, and roadsides. It grows from the lowlands to the subalpine zone. This plant is common throughout BC and is found across much of North America and into eastern Asia.

BOTANICAL DESCRIPTION

Yúla7 is a large, sturdy perennial plant that stands 4–10 feet (1–3 m) tall with single stems that are hollow, woolly, and hairy. The long-stalked leaves are very large and 8–20 inches (20–50 cm) wide, with three deeply-lobed or toothed, usually hairy, leaflets. Small white flowers are numerous in an umbrella-like cluster that is 6–12 inches (15–30.5 cm) across. The dry, oval, flattened fruits are 0.3–0.5 inch (8–13 mm) long, and are ribbed with wing-like margins.

SUSTAINABLE HARVEST AND TIMING

Shoots and flower buds can be harvested in the early spring from approximately late April to mid-May, while the plant is still small and tender. Young leaves and stalks can be harvested in May and June. Peel with caution to avoid getting the sap on your skin. The seeds can be harvested in late August to September and dehydrated for later use as a seasoning.

PLANT GIFTS

Yúla7 is similar to celery in its nutritional profile. The biggest nutritional contribution yúla7 carries is a dose of water-soluble vitamins along with its fresh and pleasant flavor. These qualities would have been a highly valued and welcome addition to Indigenous diets after a long winter without fresh plant foods.

Creamy Yúla7 and Mushroom Risotto

4–6 servings

1 cup (96 g) mushrooms of choice
2 tablespoons butter, divided in half
1–2 garlic cloves, crushed
3 cups (720 ml) water, plus more as needed
1 cup (170 g) quinoa
1 teaspoon fresh or dried yúla7 leaves
  and shoots

1 Sauté the mushrooms. If you are using wild mushrooms such as chanterelles, employ the dry sauté method by adding them to a dry nonstick pan on medium heat. As the liquid from the mushrooms releases and evaporates, add 1 tablespoon butter and the garlic and continue sautéing for 5–10 minutes. If you are using store-bought mushrooms, however, you can add them to the pan immediately with the butter and garlic and sauté for 5–10 minutes.

2 Place the water, quinoa, and mushroom sauté in a separate medium saucepan. Add in the butter and stir together while bringing to a quick boil, then simmer on low heat for 20 minutes.

3 While simmering, stir 2–3 times. Be sure to keep an eye on it so that you don't burn the bottom. Add more water as needed to keep cooking until the quinoa reaches your desired consistency.

4 Chop the dried yúla7 and sprinkle over the top.

   Serve with a side of wild greens for a highly nutritious meal.

X̲ach't

x-aw-ch-t
FIREWEED
Chamaenerion angustifolium

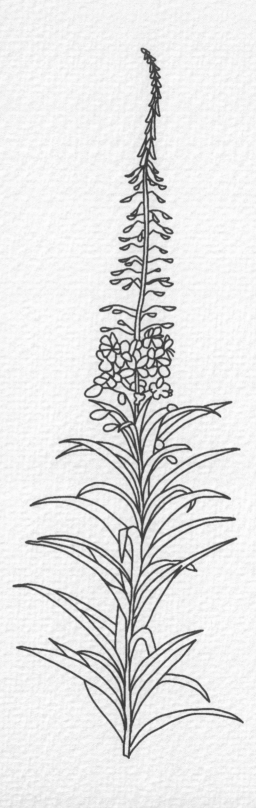

BUILDING RELATIONSHIPS

X̲ach't is one of the first plants to come back after a fire. The robust, feathery seeds can travel with the wind into disturbed sites, and are well suited for nutrient-poor and ashy soils. The magenta blooms are a sign that hunting season is starting in Squamish. In older times, the feathery seeds were incorporated into mountain goat wool to bulk it up. They were also woven into traditional Coast Salish blankets that carried rich meaning and information about one's family, village, and stature.

HABITAT

X̲ach't grows in thickets, meadows, open forests, recent forest fire sites, roadsides, and clearings. It usually grows in full sun but it can tolerate partial shade as well. It grows in soils with medium moisture from low to high elevations. X̲ach't is abundant throughout BC, and its range extends north to Alaska, Yukon, and the Northwest Territories, then down south to California and across North America to the east coast. It is globally circumboreal.

BOTANICAL DESCRIPTION

Xach't is a perennial herb that grows in large stands from a widespread rhizome-like root system. The smooth stems stand straight at 3–10 feet (1–3 m) tall. The fine-toothed leaves are 0.8–8 inches (2–20 cm) long, narrowly lanceolate, and almost stalkless as they alternate up the stems. Xach't has many deep pink to magenta flowers on the upper part of the plant. The long pink seed capsules are 1.6–4 inches (4–10 cm) long. These capsules hold the soft feather-like seeds and grow at the base of the plant while the top of the plant is still flowering.

SUSTAINABLE HARVEST AND TIMING

Xach't tends to be abundant across its range. When it is ready, it can sustain a fair amount of harvesting at various stages, based on what use you are harvesting for. In the early spring, the new shoots of xach't appear and are best harvested when they are still red and flexible. The edible leaves can be harvested throughout the growing season but are more tender in the spring. Flowers bloom from mid-to-late summer and can be harvested throughout the flowering season until they go to seed. The mature stems of xach't can be harvested in the fall, and the inner fibers of the stem processed to make a twine.

PLANT GIFTS

Xach't is anti-inflammatory, antimicrobial, and antiseptic, and can be taken as a tea or infused in honey. It can also be applied topically as an infused oil or toner. The plant is astringent and helps to reduce redness, which is great for incorporating into skincare. An oil infusion can be added to salves; if you are using a water-based recipe, an alcohol or witch-hazel infusion can be used instead. The tea can act as a mild laxative but has been used for a long time to treat digestive upsets. The shoots can be likened in taste to wild asparagus and are rich in vitamins A and C.

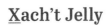

Xach't Jelly

4 cups (1280 g)

8 tightly packed cups (224 g) xach't flowers
4 cups (960 ml) water (enough to cover the flowers)
½ cup powdered pectin (about one 57-g package)
4 cups (800 g) organic cane sugar
½ cup (120 ml) lemon juice, about two lemons

1 Make a xach't tea by steeping the flowers in a pot of boiling water. Allow the tea to cool for 20 minutes.

2 Strain the liquid from the petals and reserve 3 cups (720 ml) of the tea for the jelly.

3 Bring the tea to a boil and add the pectin. Stir and dissolve well. Add the sugar and lemon juice and stir well.

4 Bring to a boil and reduce to a simmer for 15 minutes, stirring often.

5 Turn off the heat. Place the jelly in clean, hot canning jars. Wipe the tops of the jars to remove any spillage and cover with the lids.

6 Seal the lids on the jars in a hot-water bath for 10 minutes. If any lids do not seal, refrigerate and use within 3 weeks.

K̲weláwa

kwe-la-wa

NODDING ONION

Allium cernuum

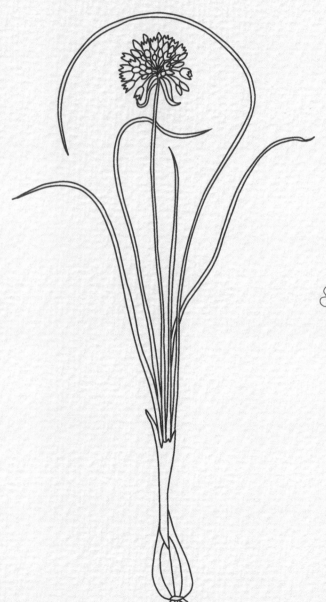

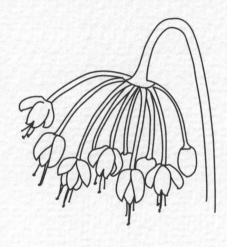

BUILDING RELATIONSHIPS

The fresh greens of k̲weláwa are fragrant in the springtime. You can often smell its spicy scent on the breeze before seeing it grow. I associate this plant with ancient Indigenous village sites. Elders have shared with me that k̲weláwa grows where Indigenous Peoples lived and cultivated their favorite plant foods to have them accessible and close to the village. I love to chew on the spring leaves of k̲weláwa to help invigorate my senses and welcome spring. The most common way this plant food was prepared in Squamish and other Indigenous communities within its range was to cook it in a pitcook, which is an underground oven that was traditionally used to cook many foods in the Squamish area and other Indigenous territories in the Pacific Northwest.

HABITAT

K̲weláwa grows at low to mid elevations in dry to mesic habitats, such as open woods or open, grassy meadows, rocky bluffs and outcrops, beaches, or other sandy sites. K̲weláwa is frequent from central BC to northern Oregon and inland to the Rockies, south to Mexico and also to the east coast of the United States. This plant thrives in a garden setting.

BOTANICAL DESCRIPTION

K̲weláwa is a pink-flowering perennial onion that grows from clustered bulbs. The flowering stem is slender and grows up to 4–20 inches (10–50 cm) tall. The slender, hairless leaves are basal and grasslike. They are shorter than the stems, and remain green as the pink to purple, nodding flower heads bloom.

SUSTAINABLE HARVEST AND TIMING

When planted in a garden, this beautiful wild onion will quickly form striking, pollinator-friendly patches through bulb division. It can be planted in full sun to partial shade and prefers good drainage. The entire plant is edible, including the bulb, foliage, and flowers. Leaves can be eaten in the early spring before the flowers come out. Bulbs can be harvested from your garden in the second year of growth, and can be used like an onion in cooking. It is recommended to divide and plant out your k̲weláwa bulbs every three years. They will also spread naturally from seed. If you wish to collect seeds, you can clip the flower heads, pour seeds into an airtight container, and store in the fridge for up to three years.

PLANT GIFTS

K̲weláwa is a bountiful food plant that has many health benefits similar to garlic and garden onions. Specifically, they are antibacterial and support immune health. A poultice of k̲weláwa leaves can be applied to the chest and throat to help ease congestion, while the bulbs and leaves can be eaten raw or cooked as a healthy addition to meals.

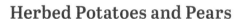

Herbed Potatoes and Pears

4–6 servings

1 tablespoon chopped fresh or dried rosemary
½ cup (50 g) chopped k̲weláwa bulbs (and leaves and stems if not too tough)
1 teaspoon sea salt
⅓ cup (80 ml) olive oil
2 tablespoons balsamic vinegar
6 medium potatoes, washed and chopped evenly
1 pear, chopped into bite-size pieces
1 tablespoon garlic powder
1 tablespoon chopped dried nettle (optional)
1 teaspoon paprika (optional)

1. Preheat the oven to 400°F (200°C).

2. In a large bowl, mix the rosemary, k̲weláwa, nettle (if using), salt, olive oil, and balsamic vinegar until well combined.

3. Add the chopped potatoes and pear to the mixture in the large bowl. Using a spatula, stir until all the potato and pear pieces are well coated with herbs and oil.

4. Spread the mixture evenly over a large baking tray lined with parchment paper.

5. Sprinkle the garlic powder and paprika (if using) over the mixture and bake for 30 minutes. Take the tray out of the oven and let cool for 10–15 minutes before serving.

Lhásem

lh-aw-sem
NORTHERN RICE ROOT
Fritillaria camschatcensis

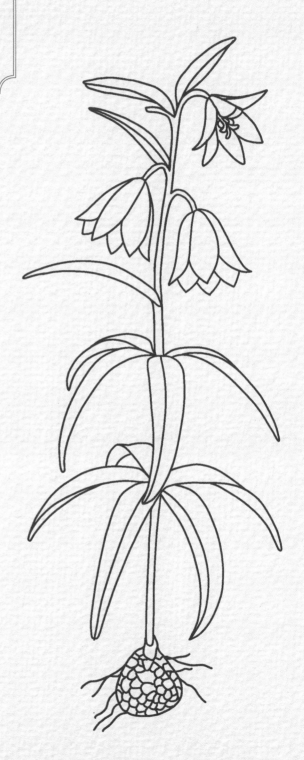

BUILDING RELATIONSHIPS

Lhásem is a special plant to me. This root vegetable was grown in intensively cultivated estuary root gardens by Indigenous communities across its range. I spent three months conducting my master's fieldwork in the Squamish Estuary, looking at restoring lhásem. I spent the days counting plant species, marking where I found lhásem growing, listening to the song of red-winged blackbirds, and watching the distant black bears emerge from the forest to dig roots along the edge of the estuary. At the end of my research, I harvested a small amount of lhásem bulbs to add to a seafood soup for a community feast. It was special to listen to people's excitement when they scooped up a lhásem bulblet in their spoon. This experience captured the joy of reconnecting with ancestral foods.

HABITAT

Lhásem grows in moist tidal flats, estuaries, meadows, open forests, rocky beaches, and streambanks from low to mid elevations and up to some subalpine meadows. Lhásem is common along the coast from Alaska through to western Washington and Oregon, extending inland occasionally to central Alaska and central BC.

BOTANICAL DESCRIPTION

Lhásem is a hairless, perennial herb that grows from a bulb consisting of several large, fleshy scales surrounded by numerous rice-like bulblets. The smooth stems are 8–31.5 inches (20–80 cm) tall, with lance-shaped leaves that are 2–4 inches (5–10 cm) long and 0.2–1 inch (0.5–2.5 cm) wide. The leaves appear in two or three main whorls of five to ten on the upper part of the stem. Flower heads have several, nodding, greenish-brown to purplish-brown or nearly black (rarely yellowish-green) bell-shaped flowers with six petals. Seed capsules are barrel-shaped, six-sided, and 0.8–1.4 inches (2–3.5 cm) long, with numerous flattened seeds inside.

SUSTAINABLE HARVEST AND TIMING

Lhásem habitat and populations have been highly impacted in many areas. This plant should not be wild harvested. Indigenous Peoples who want to renew this culturally important food can dig up the bulbs, spread the rice-grain bulblets, and replant the central bulb to encourage more plants to grow. If you want to experiment with growing this plant, it is well suited to gardens. The bulbs can be harvested in the spring or fall after the plant has gone to seed. The plants take five to seven years to germinate from seed, so you can collect seeds and scatter them around your garden area. The wait will be worth it.

PLANT GIFTS

Lhásem is a beautiful plant food and promotes a reconnection with ancestral food practices. The flavor is mild. The bulbs are an important source of carbohydrates to the traditional diets of the Indigenous Peoples in the range where it grows and was cultivated.

Lhásem Seafood Soup

approximately 2–3 quarts (2–3 L)

1 tablespoon olive oil
1 cup (130 g) diced celery
1 cup (120 g) diced onion
1 cup (115 g) diced carrot
6 garlic cloves, minced
2 teaspoons smoked paprika
Salt, to taste
2 quarts (2 L) seafood or vegetable stock
1 (15-ounce, or 425-g) can tomato sauce
1 (14-ounce, or 400-ml) can full-fat coconut milk
1½ pounds (675 g) firm white fish (halibut or cod)
Bulblets of 3–5 lhásem plants (replant main bulbs)
1 pound (450 g) shrimp or prawns, peeled and deveined
Pinch of cayenne pepper (optional)

1   Heat the olive oil in a large pot over medium heat. Add the celery, onion, and carrots and cook until soft.

2   Add in the garlic and cook for 1 minute before stirring in the smoked paprika, salt, and cayenne pepper (if using).

3   Pour in the seafood (or vegetable) stock, tomato sauce, and coconut milk, then bring to a boil before reducing to a simmer for 30 minutes.

4   Add in the fish and lhásem bulblets, cover the pot with the lid, and cook for about 8 minutes, or until the fish flakes easily and/or registers an internal temperature of 145°F (63°C). Add the shrimp and cook until the shrimp is cooked through (they should look pink and opaque).

Ts'e<u>x</u>ts'í<u>x</u>

ts-ex-ts-eh-x
STINGING NETTLE
Urtica dioica

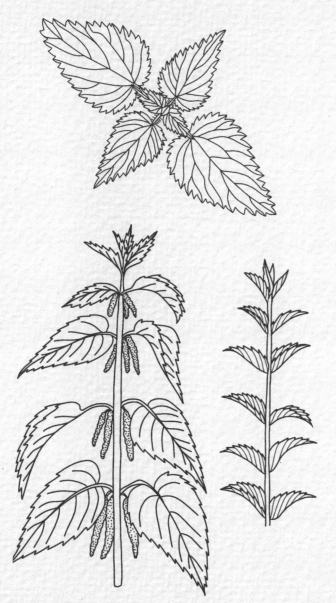

BUILDING RELATIONSHIPS

The s<u>k</u>w<u>x</u>wú7mesh name for stinging nettle, ts'e<u>x</u>ts'í<u>x</u>, comes from the root word ts'ix, meaning "singed" or "burned." My great-uncle taught me that the stinging indicates the powerful medicinal properties of this plant. He uses the fresh plant to sting himself on his arthritic joints, explaining that the sting increases blood flow and helps with swelling and pain. He learned this practice from his elders. Gloves or scissors are usually used to harvest nettles, although I've been out with many elders who don't bother with either, picking the nettles with their bare hands and hitting the fresh nettles against arthritic joints. Let's just say these elders are tough!

HABITAT

Ts'e<u>x</u>ts'í<u>x</u> grows in moist, rich soils from low to mid elevations in meadows, thickets, streambanks, and open forests. They grow in dense stands in disturbed sites such as roadsides, avalanche tracks, and barnyards. Ts'e<u>x</u>ts'í<u>x</u> is associated with historical Indigenous village sites and middens. It is found throughout BC, much of North America, and into areas of South America. Its range is very extensive, so I encourage you to do further research on whether this plant grows in your area.

WARNING: *Be sure to harvest nettles to eat fresh before they flower, as older leaves contain cystoliths, which are sharp-sided plant cells that may irritate the kidneys.*

BOTANICAL DESCRIPTION

Ts'e<u>xt</u>s'i<u>x</u> is a perennial herb with deep green leaves and tiny greenish flowers. It grows 40–120 inches (102–305 cm) tall. The stem of ts'e<u>xt</u>s'i<u>x</u> is usually less than 0.4 inch (1 cm) wide in diameter. The coarsely saw-toothed, opposite leaves are lance-shaped to oval. They have a pointed tip and a heart-shaped base and are 3–6 inches (8–15 cm) long. The flowers hang down in dense clusters of many small, whitish flowers from the leaf axil, or where the leaf stalk meets the main stem.

SUSTAINABLE HARVEST AND TIMING

Each year around late March through to mid-May is ts'e<u>xt</u>s'i<u>x</u> shoot harvesting time in Squamish. It is best harvested for eating when the young shoots are less than 1 foot (30.5 cm) tall and still have a purple tinge to the leaves, as they are at their tenderest. Nettles are very easy to grow in a garden, which is the most sustainable way to harvest this wonderful plant. The stems are gathered for fiber in September. Native butterflies such as the red admiral, comma, and small tortoiseshell butterflies lay their eggs on the leaves, and, in the fall, birds enjoy the seeds of ts'e<u>xt</u>s'i<u>x</u>. As a result, it is important to remember to leave enough of the plant for other non-human life.

PLANT GIFTS

Ts'e<u>xt</u>s'i<u>x</u> is rich in chlorophyll, vitamins, minerals, protein, and amino acids. It is considered a super food and a very nutritious spring green. The plant has antihistamine properties that help with seasonal allergies when taken as a tea. When utilized topically, either fresh or dried and infused into oil or tea, the plant carries anti-inflammatory properties that can help with sore muscles and joints. Ts'e<u>xt</u>s'i<u>x</u> is highly antioxidant, making it a nutritious food to consume to support overall immunity and health.

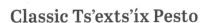

Classic Ts'e<u>xt</u>s'í<u>x</u> Pesto

1 cup (90 g)

3 cups (270 g) fresh ts'e<u>xt</u>s'í<u>x</u> leaves removed from the stems
1 cup (30g) fresh basil
2 garlic cloves, minced
¼ cup (35 g) sunflower seeds (can substitute for pine nuts, almonds, walnuts, or another nut of choice)
¼ cup (60 ml) extra virgin olive oil (for smoother consistency, add extra oil as desired)
1 tablespoon lemon juice
Pinch of sea salt, to taste
¼ cup (20 g) grated parmesan cheese (optional)

1   Blanch the fresh ts'e<u>xt</u>s'í<u>x</u> leaves for 1–2 minutes in boiling water, then drain. This will denature the stinging hairs (as will freezing, blending, or drying).

2   Add all the ingredients into a food processor or blender, and pulse until you reach your desired consistency. You will need to scrape down the sides a few times if you desire a well-blended pesto.

3   Serve over some pasta for lunch or as a creative base to your next pizza creation. You can store any leftovers in the fridge for 1 week or freeze for up to 3 months.

X̲wux̲wuk̲w'últs

xw-oh-xw-oh-kw-oh-ts

WAPATO

Sagittaria latifolia

BUILDING RELATIONSHIPS

X̲wux̲wuk̲w'últs is a plant that grows in Indigenous communities near Squamish, including the Katzie First Nation. The Squamish name x̲wux̲wuk̲w'últs is likely borrowed from a dialect of the Halkomelem language. X̲wux̲wuk̲w'últs is a root vegetable and an important source of starch in Indigenous diets. The root was cultivated and dug seasonally in marshes and wetlands. In recent years, an extensive cultivation area was uncovered during a highway project. It was found that as early as 1800 BCE, ancestors of the Katzie First Nation were managing and cultivating the wetland environment to increase the yield of this plant.

HABITAT

X̲wux̲wuk̲w'últs grows in wet or semiaquatic habitats including marshes, ponds, lakeshores, and wet ditches at mostly low elevations. Different species of x̲wux̲wuk̲w'últs occur across North America but *S. latifolia* is the species harvested in the Pacific Northwest. X̲wux̲wuk̲w'últs is infrequent in BC south of 56° N and is absent from Haida Gwaii, northern Vancouver Island, and the adjacent mainland coast. The growing range of x̲wux̲wuk̲w'últs extends south along the coast to California and east across the continent. It is more common in eastern North America, but it also occurs in Central America and into the northern regions of South America.

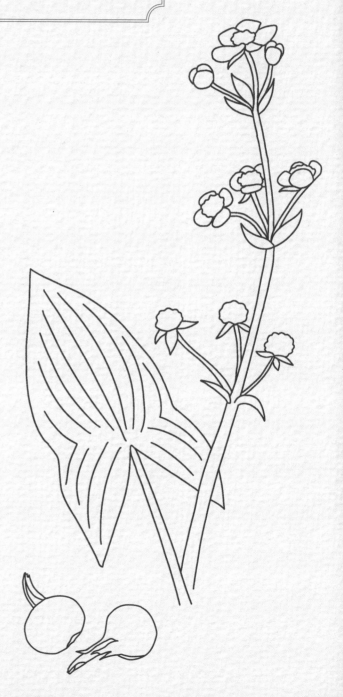

BOTANICAL DESCRIPTION

X̱wuẋwuḵw'últs is a perennial aquatic or semiaquatic plant that grows from a tuber-producing rhizome. Stems grow 8–35 inches (20–90 cm) tall. Leaves are basal; the blades of the emergent leaves are arrowhead-shaped and 2–10 inches (5–25 cm) long. The leaves have long stalks and are sheathed at the base. The blades of the submerged leaves are lance-shaped and up to 31.5 inches (80 cm) long. The flowers are white with three petals, and their stalks grow on a spike or panicle. The outer leaves, or bracts, are egg-shaped and rounded, growing 0.2–0.6 inch (5–15 mm) long. Seeds are achenes with numerous seeds in a globular cluster, and are 0.08–0.13 inch (2–3 mm) long.

SUSTAINABLE HARVEST AND TIMING

X̱wuẋwuḵw'últs is not found in Squamish and the areas where this treasured root vegetable was cultivated have been highly impacted. Consequently, this is a plant that would benefit from restoration. It is a good idea to plant your own x̱wuẋwuḵw'últs to harvest, rather than putting extra pressure on wild populations. Harvesting the tuber is best done in late August to September when the plant starts to die back. The tubers can be loosened with your hands or feet, depending on how deep the water is where they are growing. Once loosened, the tubers will float. Your harvest can be spread out across the stand; when the stands are thinned, the remaining tubers will have room to grow larger. X̱wuẋwuḵw'últs filters the water in which it grows. In highly contaminated areas, it can accumulate heavy metals, so know the history of your growing or harvesting site.

PLANT GIFTS

X̱wuẋwuḵw'últs is a beloved root vegetable that was cultivated and intensively harvested, enjoyed, and traded. This plant food supported whole communities of people. The tubers were an important source of carbohydrates to Indigenous diets that were lacking in them. They are also rich in protein, vitamins, and minerals. The plant food is important for Indigenous communities who are renewing its cultivation and all the associated knowledge and experience that comes with welcoming an ancestral food back onto the feast table.

X̱wuẋwuḵw'últs Mash

2–4 servings

1 pound (450 g) x̱wuẋwuḵw'últs tubers, washed and peeled
1 cup (240 ml) milk (or unsweetened nondairy alternative)
¼ cup (57 g) butter
1 teaspoon salt, plus a pinch for the boiling water
1 teaspoon dried thyme
½ teaspoon black pepper

1 Place the x̱wuẋwuḵw'últs tubers into a large pot and fill it three-quarters with water, enough to immerse the tubers. Season the water with salt and boil the tubers for approximately 30 minutes, or until tender.

2 Mash the x̱wuẋwuḵw'últs in a large bowl (or in the pot after draining). Once you have thoroughly mashed the tubers, add the milk and butter. Mix the ingredients together.

3 Add the salt, thyme, and pepper and mix well.

X̲et'tánay

xet-tan-eye
WILD GINGER
Asarum caudatum

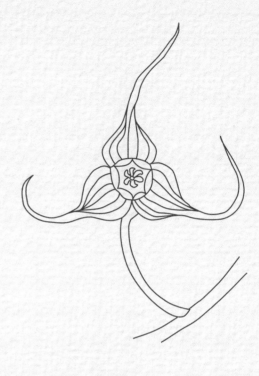

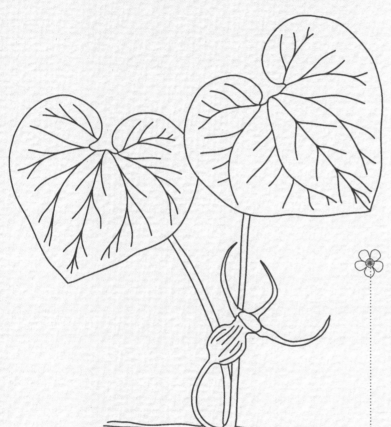

 BUILDING RELATIONSHIPS

X̲et'tánay is one of those plants that I was so excited
to find for the first time! It has such a gorgeous
and unique bloom. I found it growing in the forest
when I was on a cedar bark harvesting trip with
my immediate and extended family. We were out
looking for good cedar trees to harvest bark from
and I noticed the dark green, heart-shaped leaves
in a large patch on the forest floor. The closer I
got, I realized this was x̲et'tánay! I got down on
the ground and lifted the leaves looking for the

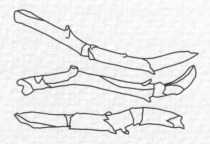

WARNING: *Never tincture the plant in alcohol
or infuse the root in vinegar, as this concentrates
the plant compounds that are harmful to us in
higher concentrations. Please read this section
carefully as there is more information on
consuming x̲et'tánay safely.*

unique flowers. The flowers have three dark purple to brown petals that thin into tendrils at the ends. They are beautiful and different from any other flower I've seen growing in this region. The dark green leaves might hide the deep purple-brown flower so it takes some care and attention to notice xet'tánay growing low to the ground.

HABITAT

Xet'tánay grows in moist, nutrient-rich soils in shaded forest sites at low to mid elevations. It grows frequently in southern BC, and south into California, Idaho, and Montana.

BOTANICAL DESCRIPTION

Xet'tánay is a perennial herb that grows from extensive rhizomes forming large mats, with the stems rooting freely. Leaves are 1–4 inches (2.5–10 cm) long and 2–6 inches (5–15 cm) wide, have long stalks, are heart-shaped and shiny, and have leaf veins covered in fine hair. The solitary, bell-shaped, purplish-brown flowers have three flaring lobes that are long and pointed. The fruiting capsules are spherical and fleshy with several egg-like seeds.

SUSTAINABLE HARVEST AND TIMING

This is a beautiful and unique plant and I have planted xet'tánay from native plant nurseries into my garden with great success. The leaves, stems, and rhizomes can be harvested in the spring or summer and dried or used fresh to make a mild tea or water infusion. They can also be eaten fresh in small amounts. Xet'tánay contains aristolochic acid, which is known to be toxic at high concentrations. Aristolochic acid is not very water-soluble, but if ingesting it you should only consume diluted infusions. People with preexisting kidney ailments should not ingest this plant.

PLANT GIFTS

Though this plant has a long history of use in many Indigenous communities, it needs to be handled by someone who knows how to prepare it safely, or it should be avoided. The leaves and stems of xet'tánay are the most fragrant and flavorful parts of the plant. The rhizomes are also fragrant but are considered mildly toxic and are not safe to consume in large amounts. Xet'tánay has been used in Squamish as a treatment for tuberculosis. The leaves were chewed and the juice swallowed. There are other Indigenous communities that infuse the plant into a tea to ease stomach upset, as well as use the plant topically as a poultice for treating arthritis. On the other hand, because this plant contains aristolochic acid, which is known to be toxic at high concentrations, it is worth doing your own research to develop your comfort with ingesting xet'tánay. Even if you just taste a small piece of the stem, leaf, or root, it is a refreshing treat.

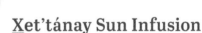

Xet'tánay Sun Infusion

1 quart (1 L)

3–5 fresh-picked xet'tánay leaves and stems
1 quart (1 L) filtered water

1   Roughly chop the leaves and stems and place them in a clean, quart-sized (1 L) jar.

2   Pour the filtered water over the xet'tánay and let it infuse in the sun for 30–60 minutes.

3   Strain the plant ingredients out of the water. Enjoy the citrusy flavor with an ice cube on a sunny day.

Schi7i7áý

sch-eh-eh-eye

WILD STRAWBERRY

Fragaria chiloensis,
F. virginiana, **and** *F. vesca*

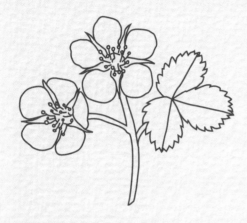

BUILDING RELATIONSHIPS

Schi7i7áý carries so much flavor in such a tiny fruit. When you come upon a patch of the tiny red, sweet schi7i7áý creeping along the ground, hidden under green-lobed leaves, it truly is like finding treasure. The name schi7i7áý can refer to different species of wild strawberry, but all schi7i7áý can be eaten and utilized in the same ways. I can recall finding patches of schi7i7áý at forest edges at mid elevations around Squamish, crawling around inspecting under leaves for the small but delicious fruits. I imagine my Squamish ancestors doing the same, as these have been a favorite food for generations.

WARNING: *Use schi7i7áý leaves fresh, or dried but not wilted, as hydrogen cyanide is released by the wilting leaves as a defense for the plant and can be harmful.*

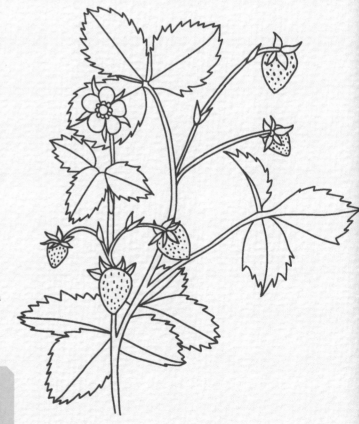

HABITAT

Schi7i7áý refers to three different species. *Fragaria chiloensis* grows in mesic to dry dunes, sandy/gravelly beaches, and rocky bluffs and islets along marine shorelines. It grows in strictly coastal areas from Alaska to California, but also in areas of South America and Hawaii. *F. virginiana* and *F. vesca* grow in dry to moist meadows, grassy slopes, thickets, riparian areas, forest edges, open forests, clearings, and roadsides, as well as in low to subalpine elevations. They appear frequently from Alaska, south through BC to California, and eastward across the continent.

BOTANICAL DESCRIPTION

Schi7i7áý is a perennial herb with a scaly rhizome and long, slender leafless runners that grow from the main plant and root along the way. These runners are called stolons, and they are often green to red in color. The long-stalked leaves grow at the base of the plant and have three coarsely toothed leaflets, similar to cultivated strawberries. The small white flowers have five petals. The fruit are small and red, elongated or spherical in shape, and 0.4–0.6 inch (1–1.5 cm) across.

SUSTAINABLE HARVEST AND TIMING

The leaves can be harvested in the spring before the berries from the schi7i7áý ripen in the spring or early summer. They take quite a long time to harvest given the size of the fruit, so they are best eaten fresh, right as they are harvested. However, if you have the self-control to collect enough to incorporate the berries into recipes, they are wonderful in jams, pies, and fruit leather. In some areas the schi7i7áý may be declining, so be sure to look for plentiful patches of the plant—or better yet, grow it in your garden!

PLANT GIFTS

Schi7i7áý carries many gifts, including the tasty fruits that are packed with beneficial nutrients, such as flavonoids and ellagic acid, which is strongly antioxidant. The astringent leaves can be made into a facial toner or facial steam. They can also be used to make a vitamin C-rich tea for upset stomachs and to help keep colds at bay.

Schi7i7áý-Leaf Facial Steam

1 use

1 quart (1 L) boiling water
½ cup (15 g) dried schi7i7áý leaves
½ cup (20 g) dried lavender
2–4 drops of lavender or rosemary essential oil or other essential oil of choice (optional)

1   Carefully pour the boiling water over the schi7i7áý leaves and lavender in a heat-safe bowl.

2   Add 2–4 drops of essential oil (or less, if so inclined).

3   Let the water cool slightly, then place your face over the steam. Put a towel over your head and the bowl to concentrate the steam on your face. Stay here for 5–15 minutes and then cleanse, tone, and moisturize. Enjoy the calming benefits of the schi7i7áý leaves and the calming scent of lavender.

Si7semáchxw

say-sem-ah-ch-xw

YARROW

Achillea millefolium

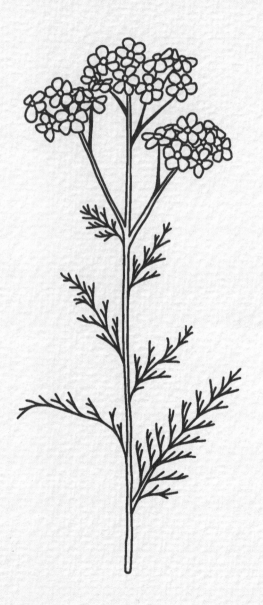

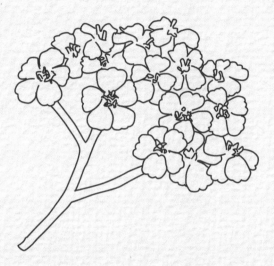

 BUILDING RELATIONSHIPS

Si7semáchxw is an incredible healer. This plant has been valued for its medicinal and culinary applications for millennia. I first learned about its anti-inflammatory properties when I was working in Kingcome Inlet, home to the Musgamakw Dzawada'enuxw First Nation who are part of the broader Kwakwaka'wakw people. Two elders asked me to harvest a big bag of yarrow leaves for them. They told me they used them as a bath tea to help relieve aching joints and sore muscles. In Squamish, the leaves were chewed to help ease toothaches, or steeped and prepared as a tea to calm the stomach.

HABITAT

Si7semáchxw grows in mesic to dry sites including coastal bluffs, meadows, grasslands, rocky slopes, and open forests. Si7semáchxw is common and widespread throughout BC, north to Alaska, Yukon, and the Northwest Territories, and throughout Florida, Texas, California, and into Mexico.

BOTANICAL DESCRIPTION

Si7semáchxw is a perennial herb that grows from a rhizome and has tall, slender stems that can be 4–40 inches (10–101 cm) tall. The aromatic, feathery leaves have a fernlike appearance and are pinnately dissected. The flower heads consist of a flat, round-topped cluster of tiny whitish flowers, usually numbering from fifteen to forty.

SUSTAINABLE HARVEST AND TIMING

Si7semáchxw season arrives in the warmer months. The plant is usually in bloom from May to September. The fragrant, feathery leaves are present earlier in the season starting from the month of April. This plant is easy to grow in a garden setting; consequently, this is the most sustainable way to harvest the plant. When harvesting the flower, be sure not to take the first you find. Look at the overall size of the stand you intend to harvest from and spread out your harvest, and do not take more than half the stand. I use scissors or clippers when harvesting so that the roots remain intact underground, ensuring that the plant returns year after year.

PLANT GIFTS

When you pick a leaf from si7semáchxw and crush it between your fingers, the fragrant oils are released and the scent is earthy and sensuous.

I love this plant: its scent and healing properties, along with the fact that it is very easy to grow in a garden, make it a wonderful botanical ingredient to have on hand. The leaves of the plant can be dried and powdered and used as a styptic to stop bleeding. They are also anti-inflammatory and can be added to baths, infused oils, salves, and ointments to promote healing of mild burns and skin irritations. The leaves can be steeped and prepared into a tea or used to flavor your favorite dish. The leaves of yarrow contain many beneficial nutrients including calcium, magnesium, niacin, phosphorous protein, riboflavin, vitamins A and C, zinc, and more.

Si7semáchxw Bath Tea

enough for 1 bath

1 bunch dried yarrow leaves and flowers

1   Place a blend of dried yarrow leaves and flowers (see drying botanicals on page 46) in a square of cheesecloth and securely tie it off. I tend to use about 2 cups (109 g) of flowers and leaves.

2   Draw a nice hot bath (but not too hot) and let the bag steep in the bathwater for 5 to 10 minutes before you bathe. Keep the bag in the water to enhance the scent and topical benefits of the plant.

Blend with other aromatic plants, such as lavender or coastal sage, for a different sensory experience.

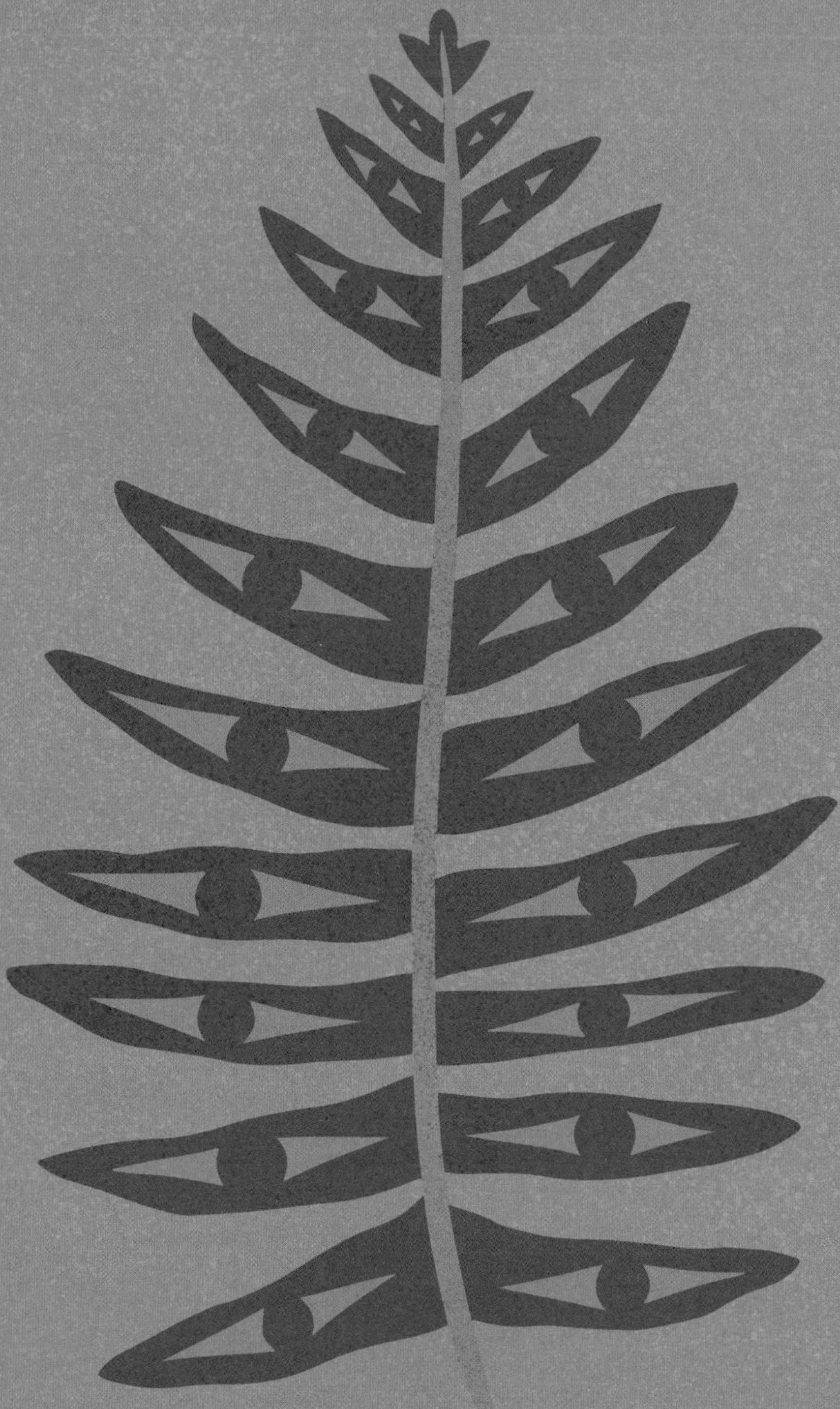

FERNS, HORSETAILS, LICHENS & SEAWEEDS

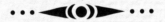

Mimts'

BEARD LICHEN

Usnea longissima
(Squamish name may
also refer to *Alectoria
sarmentosa*)

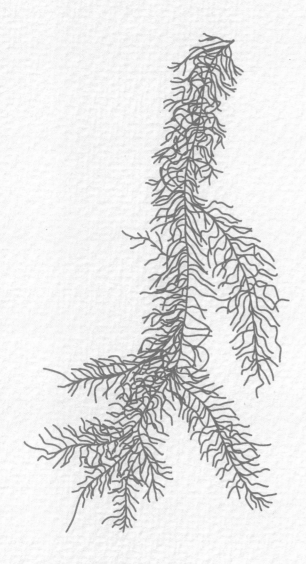

 BUILDING RELATIONSHIPS

Mimts' is characteristic of rainforests in the Pacific
Northwest. A lichen that hangs from moss-covered
tree branches, it signifies the cleanliness of the
air. The way it sways in the wind brings a calm
feeling to me, even when I close my eyes and think
of it. Lichen is a symbiotic organism comprised of
fungi and algae that come together to create
a unique lifeform. The fungi create the structure,
and the algae photosynthesize. During the start
of the COVID-19 pandemic, I felt drawn to mimts',
as I knew of its highly antibacterial and antiviral
properties. I also found a sense of deep calm
visualizing a place in Squamish Territory where
mimts' grows extensively. I decided to create
some wellness products—like a gentle hand soap,
a calming room mist, and a nourishing hand
balm—that all incorporated mimts' as a way
of connecting more deeply to this lichen.

HABITAT

Mimts' grows on the branches and bark of trees, usually conifers. Some species of *Usnea,* including *Usnea longissima,* grow longer and hang down from the conifer branches like billowing curtains. *Usnea longissima* grows in coastal temperate rainforests from Alaska into Northern California.

BOTANICAL DESCRIPTION

Mimts' is a large, pale-yellowish to green hanging hair lichen that grows 6–40 inches (15–100 cm) or longer. It has a long central strand with many smaller side branches. The white central cord is characteristic of this species and helps distinguish it from other beard lichens that have colored cords. Witch's hair and old man's beard lichens (*Alectoria* spp.) lack central cords.

SUSTAINABLE HARVEST AND TIMING

Mimts', like other lichens, grows very slowly, so the most sustainable way to harvest it is from fallen branches on the forest floor. In forests where mimts' is growing abundantly, this will not be difficult to do. Branches fall down during windstorms; I have often found many mimts'-laden branches on the ground after a big windstorm in Squamish. Mimts' can be harvested year-round.

PLANT GIFTS

Mimts' is highly antibacterial and antiviral, and thus has historically lent itself as a medicine for treating many ailments. Mimts' can be dried and powdered and used as first aid for cuts or scrapes.

If infused in oil or tinctured in alcohol, usnic acid (one of the main compounds found in mimts') carries antibacterial and antiviral properties that promote wound healing. Once an infusion is made with mimts', it can be added to topical treatments as well as internal treatments. I encourage the reader to research this powerful medicinal lichen to learn more.

Mimts' First Aid Powder

approximately 2 tablespoons

5 handfuls or bundles mimts', harvested from fallen branches

1 Clean the mimts' of any bark or other debris.

2 Place the mimts' in a coffee grinder (used for plants only) and grind into a powder.

3 Remove any fibrous strands that are left.

4 Sift the mimts' powder through a fine-mesh sieve.

5 Pour the powdered mimts' into a clean, dry glass jar or tin and store in a cool, dry place, or add it to your first aid kit.

6 Apply the powder directly to cuts in order to slow bleeding and benefit from the plant's antibacterial properties.

   If you have the whole plant, you can remove the twigs and pour boiling water over the plant in a heat-safe bowl. Wait for it to cool, then apply the still-hot lichen directly to skin.

Sx̱ém̓x̱em

sx-uhm-ex-uhm

COMMON HORSETAIL

Equisetum arvense

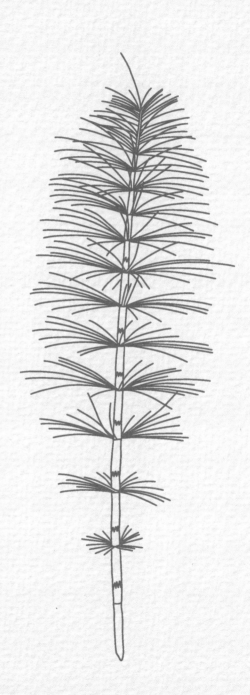

BUILDING RELATIONSHIPS

I remember learning about sx̱ém̓x̱em in my plant taxonomy class in university because of how widespread this plant is. Horsetails are some of the most ancient plants on the planet; some say they can be considered living fossils, which is pretty amazing! Additionally, I always think about the benefits for hair and nails when I see this plant. The silica is such a great ingredient for strengthening hair and nails when applied topically or taken internally, either as a spring green or a tea.

WARNING: *The green stems of some horsetail species contain thiaminase, an enzyme that depletes thiamine or vitamin B1 stores in the body. As a result, the green stems should not be ingested fresh and should be used in moderation when dried. People with conditions including diabetes, gout, and kidney disorders should seek medical advice before using.*

164

HABITAT

Sx̱émx̱em grows in moist to wet sites including forests, meadows, swamps, alpine seepage areas, and along roadsides in dense patches. Sx̱émx̱em is very widespread from Alaska along the entire coastline of the Pacific Northwest into California and across most of North America. It can also be found in Greenland, Eurasia, north Africa, and New Zealand.

BOTANICAL DESCRIPTION

Sx̱émx̱em is a perennial that grows from a hairy, tuber-bearing rhizome. The jointed, hollow-ridged stems of the sterile part of the plant grow from 4–32 inches (10–80 cm) tall and 0.1–0.2 inch (2.5–5 mm) thick, with branches growing in regular whorls around the stem. The fertile stems are shorter, unbranched, and brown to yellow in color, and are visually similar to succulents. The fertile stems appear in the spring before the taller sterile stems.

SUSTAINABLE HARVEST AND TIMING

Sx̱émx̱em grows abundantly across its wide range, so you generally don't have to worry about overharvesting this plant for personal use. The early fertile spring shoots are edible. The sterile stems can be harvested throughout the growing season to be infused for topical use. In a pinch, the mature stems make great nail files or pot scrubbers.

PLANT GIFTS

You can make a tea infusion to sip in moderation; my Squamish ancestors drank the water from the hollow stems as a spring tonic and ate the fresh spring fertile shoots. Sx̱émx̱em is rich in silica, which helps support nail, bone, and hair health when eaten or applied topically. Try out this nail-strengthening cuticle oil that can be applied to nails and hair to enhance strength and luster.

Sx̱émx̱em Strong Nails Cuticle Oil

2 cups (480 ml)

2 cups (480 ml) organic jojoba or castor oil, or a blend of the two
1 cup (140 g) dried sx̱émx̱em
15–30 drops lavender or peppermint essential oil (optional)

1   Pour water in the bottom pot of your double boiler, being careful not to have the water touching the bottom of the top pot. Place the top pot over the bottom and ensure it is dry.

2   Add the oil and dried sx̱émx̱em to the top pot of the double boiler and infuse the ingredients over medium heat for 2–4 hours.

3   Take the double boiler off the heat and allow the cuticle oil to cool. If you would like the cuticle oil to be more concentrated, you can let it sit somewhere to cool overnight.

4   Strain out the sx̱émx̱em. Add the essential oil if using. Store the oil in a clean, dry glass bottle with a dropper or pump top.

5   Apply a drop to your cuticles and massage into your nails daily. Apply it to the ends of your hair too!

This infused oil will last for up to 6 months if all of the plant material is strained out. It will last even longer if it is stored in the fridge.

Tl'esíp

tl-e-say-p
LICORICE FERN
Polypodium glycyrrhiza

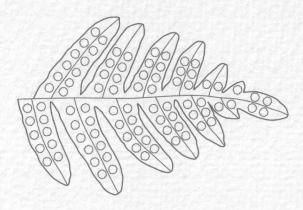

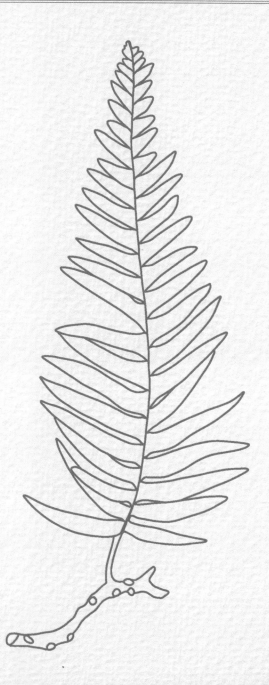

BUILDING RELATIONSHIPS

Tl'esíp unfurls with bright-green fronds in the fall, the opposite of most botanical life in the region. Squamish Peoples have chewed on the rhizomes during ceremonies and celebrations to keep their singing voices strong. The licorice flavor of tl'esíp is one of my favorite forest flavors, fresh or dried. There are many medicines that have been prepared with tl'esíp for topical and internal ailments in Squamish. For example, it is a key ingredient in a drink to help calm stomach upset.

HABITAT

Tl'esíp is commonly epiphytic and grows on the mossy branches of deciduous trees, mainly bigleaf maple in the Squamish area but also red alder, Sitka spruce, and other trees elsewhere on the coast. It occurs on moist, mossy bedrock slabs, outcrops, boulders, and fallen logs. It is frequently found in coastal BC, north to southeast Alaska, south to California, and inland to southern BC and Idaho.

BOTANICAL DESCRIPTION

Tl'esíp is a small-to-medium fern that can be evergreen, but sends out new growth in the fall. The fronds grow up to 4–27 inches (10–70 cm) long (but often much shorter) and 0.8–6 inches (2–15 cm) wide from a reddish-brown, licorice-flavored scaly rhizome. The frond is lance-shaped, and the once-pinnate leaflets are 1.2 inches (3 cm) or longer with pointed tips. The sori are roundish and can be found in one row on either side of the main vein.

SUSTAINABLE HARVEST AND TIMING

Tl'esíp is slow growing, and its rhizomes creep and expand under the moss-covered substrate. Therefore, it is important to pat the moss back into place once the rhizome segment has been removed. It is best to take the fresh, new green growth on the rhizomes and leave the older, woodier rhizome systems in place. You can also grow tl'esíp in your garden by planting it with some buried rocks. The fern reproduces through spores carried on the wind, so you can also help spread the spores around when you harvest the rhizomes.

PLANT GIFTS

Tl'esíp has a long history of being an important medicine for sore throats and colds, and to support ceremony. The rhizomes are thought to contain a compound called polypodoside, which is 600 times sweeter than table sugar. I have powdered the rhizome for use as a sweetener and have definitely noticed the burst of sweetness when the plant hits my tongue. Licorice fern also has an enzyme called thiaminase, which at high levels can deplete vitamin B, so use this plant in moderation.

Cranberry–Tl'esíp Biscotti

10–12 biscotti

3 eggs
1 tablespoon balsamic vinegar
1 tablespoon apple cider vinegar
1 tablespoon vanilla extract
¼ cup (60 ml) honey
1 teaspoon ground cinnamon
2 tablespoons ground dried or fresh tl'esíp root
⅓ cup (70 g) cane sugar
1 cup (235 g) dried cranberries
2 cups (250 g) all-purpose flour
1 teaspoon baking powder

1 Preheat the oven to 300°F (150°C).

2 Place the eggs, balsamic vinegar, apple cider vinegar, vanilla, and honey in a blender. Blend on low for 30 seconds and set aside.

3 Place the remaining ingredients in a large bowl and mix with a spatula.

4 Pour in the liquid ingredients from the blender and mix until a batter forms.

5 Roll out the dough on a large baking sheet lined with parchment paper with a rolling pin.

6 Use your hands to form the dough lengthwise into an even log. Flatten the top and sides a little if needed to make it even.

7 Bake for 35 minutes and let cool for 15 minutes.

8 Using a serrated bread knife, cut the loaf into ¾-inch (2 cm) slices. You should now have around 10–12 biscotti pieces.

9 Spread the sliced pieces around the baking pan, flat sides up, and bake for another 20 minutes, flipping them over at the 10-minute mark. Doing this ensures they firm up and become crispy.

Lhék'es

lh-uh-k-es

RED LAVER

Pyropia abbottiae

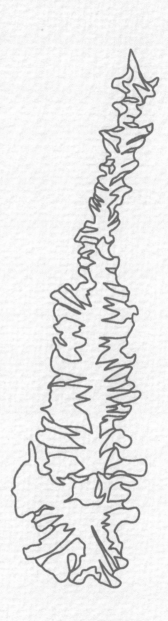

BUILDING RELATIONSHIPS

The first time I harvested lhék'es was in Kwakwakw'wakw territory while learning from elders of the region. I still smile to this day recalling the feeling of being a part of that harvesting trip. We harvested lhék'es under the guidance of Kwakwakw'wakw elders and learned how to process the lhék'es into dried cakes for later use in ceremony and trade.

HABITAT

Lhék'es can be found growing on semi-exposed to exposed rocks in the low to mid intertidal zone. It is found in Alaska, along the coast of the Pacific Northwest, and down to Mexico.

BOTANICAL DESCRIPTION

Lhék'es is a red alga that ranges in color from brown to purplish to nearly black. It is thin and nearly transparent. The thallus (body) of lhék'es is one cell thick, and can be up to 19.6 inches (50 cm) long and 2 inches (5 cm) wide.

SUSTAINABLE HARVEST AND TIMING

Lhék'es is harvested early in the morning to allow for ample drying time. Generally it is picked in the spring when the new growth is fresh, but this varies across Indigenous communities. Spreading out your harvest is important and it is recommended to harvest at a low tide, pull the lhék'es from the rocks, shake it out to release any little critters that may be holding on, and then dry it in cakes as soon as possible. To dry lhék'es, you spread it out into square cakes approximately 1–1.5 feet (30–46 cm) on dry rocks, ideally in a location facing the sun and wind. Once one side of the seaweed cake is dry, you can flip it over and dry the other side.

PLANT GIFTS

Lhék'es has a long history of being gifted during ceremonies including potlatches, which are large ceremonial gatherings where Indigenous communities in the Pacific Northwest come together and share in a feast, dancing and singing. Wealth is redistributed and activities concerning trade, law, and economy are carried out. This food is highly nutritious; seaweeds in this family are widely considered to be health foods, as they are rich in protein, carbohydrates, minerals, and vitamins. Most notably, lhék'es contains high levels of iodine, vitamin A, and salt. To give an idea of the widespread appreciation and use of this food, lhék'es is the same seaweed that is called nori in Japan.

Lhék'es and Mint Rejuvenating Bath Soak

enough for 6–8 baths

1 cup (397g) pink Himalayan bath salts
1 cup (230 g) Epsom salts
1 cup (230 g) Dead Sea salts
½ cup (74 g) powdered dry mint or peppermint leaves
¼ cup (37 g) lhék'es powder
5–20 drops spearmint or peppermint essential oil

1 Measure out all the ingredients, except for the essential oil, into a large bowl.

2 Mix the dry ingredients together well with a fork or whisk until both powders are blended and coat the salt.

3 Scent with 5–20 drops of chosen essential oil. Start with less and add more if you prefer a stronger scent. Mix well.

4 Bottle the bath soak powder in one large airtight container or smaller containers.

5 Sprinkle approximately ½ cup (121 g) of salts into a hot bath and enjoy!

CONCLUSION

I hope you have enjoyed this book and the information I have shared. I encourage you to continue to learn, gather your own experiences, and build your knowledge of and relationships with plants. Plants offer so many teachings and so many ways to support health and wellness. It is a lifelong learning that develops over seasons and many hours spent on the land observing, connecting to, growing, harvesting, and processing plants. I will leave you with some final reflections.

 ## Next Steps

There are many resources out there to learn more about all aspects of plants, from their botany and ecology to their cultural contexts. I encourage you to collect some key resources, such as plant field guides, a field notebook to record information about the timing of different stages in a plant's life cycle, and information on the location of particular plants. Having notes from previous seasons can be so helpful in building connections to the places that you frequent on the land season after season. It is also nice to record the other life you notice when you are out—the birds and insects that interact with the plants, and the other animals that are also in relationship with particular plants and places. Rebuilding connections to the land and to the histories of botanical interrelationships that we all carry is a way of healing and strengthening ourselves, and can become our motivation for giving back to the land and advocating for living in sustainable and environmentally minded ways.

Good Frame of Mind and Heart

My great-auntie Eva told me that when we are creating something, whatever we are carrying in our hearts and whatever feelings we have go into what we are creating. If we are making a meal for loved ones or making a medicine to support health, it is important to stop and feel into our own state of mind and heart.

To me, this is a culturally grounded teaching in mindfulness and self-awareness. It is a pause that can not only help us to consider the greater good and purpose of our actions, but also assess our own personal state of mind. I know from experience that stopping to check in with myself, to bring awareness to my mind, body, and heart, can help to reset and to identify and address any tensions, hard feelings, or distractions that may be present.

Author and mindfulness teacher Tara Brach writes about the sacred pause, which is the opportunity we all have (but that often evades us for a myriad of reasons) to take a purposeful and mindful pause between a trigger and a response. This pause may make the difference between acting out of anger, defensiveness, or hurt, and can facilitate changing rote responses to align more with the version of ourselves we wish to be. To apply the sacred pause when we are creating something to support our own or another's well-being, we can also consider the teaching my aunt shared with me: that what we are thinking and what we are feeling in our hearts can go into what we are creating, which gives us the opportunity to mindfully decide how we want to hold space for creating. This may mean coming back to it later or taking time to care for yourself in order to reset.

This teaching is one that I have heard from many elders since, and is rooted in gentle accountability and self-awareness of how we are in relationship with ourselves and others. I carry these teachings in my heart as I continue to rebuild my relationships with and knowledge of plants. It is always a beautiful reminder to slow down and connect with my heart when I am working with plants.

Continuity

My ancestral name Styawat was given to me by my great-uncle Chester Thomas from my Snuneymuxw (Nanaimo First Nation) side of my family. It translates to "the wind that blows away the clouds and brings the sun." He blanketed me with this name to protect me, to strengthen my identity, and to bravely practice the culture he was abused for in his residential school years.

My great-uncle Chester had huge hands, the creases always lined with earth from his garden and charcoal from his smokehouse. He and my great-auntie Eva had a home along the Nanaimo River, and it was one of my havens growing up. Their home smelled of woodsmoke and felt like a warm hug. I remember looking out a window that faced the back of their house; in my childhood memory, the golden fields of long grasses seemed to span forever into the horizon. These early visits ignited a spark in my spirit. I knew this by how my heart felt as a child, but I didn't understand it in a cerebral way until much later in my life. I add this reflection as a reminder of how our lives and stories are made up of moments: time spent with loved ones, meals shared together, the love bestowed upon us by those closest to us in our lives. Part of renewing land-based practices is both honoring those who have walked these lands before us and reigniting embers of knowledge, land-based connection, and wellness for those yet to come.

Being a Good Future Ancestor

I heard this phrase a few years ago, and it took me a little while to understand what it meant. I had an *aha!* moment when I realized that I will be someone's ancestor. The life I am living now will have a ripple effect and carry through generations to come. Every teaching I gain and each experience I have that brings me closer to the land and to my culture is also my responsibility to carry in a good way and to pass on with love and care.

It is too easy today not to look beyond our own existence, our own individual needs and desires. But when I think of my life on a greater continuum, I think about the legacy I want to leave and the type of world I wish to contribute to. I believe we can all reflect on this and consider the questions: What do we want our grandchildren's grandchildren to inherit? What teachings and stories of our lives do we want to carry on in the generations to come? To me, these are inseparable from the question: What kind of earth do we want to see generations from now, and how can we act now to contribute to that?

I will leave you with these reflections, and I thank you from the bottom of my heart for engaging with and reading this offering. I hope it brings you closer to the natural world and that these pages support your own botanical relationships.

BOTANICAL GLOSSARY

Achene: A small, dry, one-seeded fruit with a thin wall that remains closed at maturity. An example is a sunflower.

Alpine zone: A region that occurs above the treeline and below the snowline on temperate and tropical mountains.

Alternate leaves: An alternate leaf arrangement is one where there is one leaf per plant node, and the leaves alternate sides.

Basal: Leaves, or other plant parts, that are situated or attached at the base of a plant.

Bloom: A whitish powdery coating on the surface of certain fruits and leaves.

Bog: An ecosystem that is characterized by nutrient-poor substrates such as acidic, saturated peatmoss, and scattered or clumped, stunted conifer trees amongst sphagnum mosses and ericaceous shrubs.

Cambium: A thin layer between the xylem and phloem of most vascular plants that gives rise to new cells and is responsible for new seasonal, or secondary, growth.

Circumboreal: Refers to plants found growing in regions of North America and Eurasia close to the Arctic.

Compound leaf: Leaves with depressions along the leaf margin that are so deep they split the leaf blades into leaflets.

Deciduous: Trees and shrubs that, unlike evergreens, lose their leaves and become dormant during the winter.

Dissected: A leaf that is deeply divided into numerous segments.

Dome: A flower having the shape of a dome. It is another descriptor for an umbel.

Drupelet: A single small subdivision which makes up the outer layer of certain fruit such as blackberries or raspberries. Can also refer to a singular drupe.

Edges: Refers to the boundary of two habitats. This could be the edge of a forest or edge of a meadow, etc. This helps in predicting the habitat where certain plants will be found growing.

Epiphytic: A plant that grows on tree branches or cliffs that derives nutrients from the air and rain.

Inflorescence: A group or a cluster of flowers arranged on a stem that is composed of a main branch or a complicated arrangement of branches.

Lance: A leaf or other plant part that is spear-shaped and usually elongated.

Lanceolate: A leaf shaped like a lance head and that is narrow and tapering to a pointed end. It can be lancelike or lance-shaped.

Leaf margins: The edge of a leaf. Can be serrated, smooth, lobed, or deeply toothed.

Leaflet: One of the divisions of a compound leaf.

Linear: A leaf or plant part that is very narrow in relation to its length, with the sides mostly parallel.

Lobed: Leaves, petals, or seeds that have lobes or divisions extending less than halfway to the middle of the base.

Margins: Refers to the perimeter of a leaf from top to bottom.

Mesic: Refers to plants that grow in areas of medium water supply or soil moisture.

Montane: Ecosystems found on the slopes of mountains. The alpine climate in these regions strongly affects the ecosystem because temperatures fall as elevation increases, which impacts the plants growing in these regions.

Node: The points on a stem where the buds, leaves, and branching twigs originate.

Open: Refers to an ecosystem or growing area for plants that is reasonably open and lets light in through the canopy.

Opposite leaves: Two leaves that grow from the stem at the same level, or at the same node, on opposite sides of the stem.

Panicle: A panicle is a branched raceme in which each branch has more than one flower.

Petiole: The stalk of a leaf.

Phloem: Specialized vascular tissue in a plant that conduct foods that are made in the leaves during the process of photosynthesis to all other parts of the plant.

Pinnate: A compound leaf structure with a feather-like formation of leaflets arranged either in pairs or alternating along the main stem.

Pome: A fleshy fruit, such as an apple or pear, that consists of an outer fleshy layer that is thick plus a central core that usually has five seeds enclosed in a capsule.

Raceme: A simple inflorescence in which the flowers are borne on short stalks of about equal length at equal distances along the stem.

Rhizome: A modified subterranean, or underground, plant stem that sends out roots and shoots from its nodes. Rhizomes are also called creeping rootstalks or, more simply, rootstalks.

Runner: A slender trailing stem that produces roots and sometimes erect shoots at its nodes. Also called a stolon.

Sori: Brownish or yellowish round clusters of spore-producing structures (sporangia) usually located on the lower surface of fern leaves. Known as *sorus* in the singular.

Stand: A group or growth of tall plants or trees.

Stolon: See Runner.

Substrate: The surface on which a plant or fungus lives (e.g., soil, rock, tree branch, etc.).

Suckers: Vigorous vertical shoots that grow from the roots or lower main stem. They take energy away from the main plants and can be pruned back in plant management.

Thallus: The plant body in algae, fungi, or mosses that is not differentiated into stems, leaves, or roots.

Umbel: A cluster of flowers made up of several short stalks that spread from a common point, resembling the ribs of an umbrella.

Whorl: A ring of plant parts borne at the same level on an axis (e.g., leaves or floral parts).

Woody: Refers to plants that have hard stems.

Xylem: Refers to a type of vascular tissue that is responsible for conducting water throughout the body of a plant.

Types of Leaves

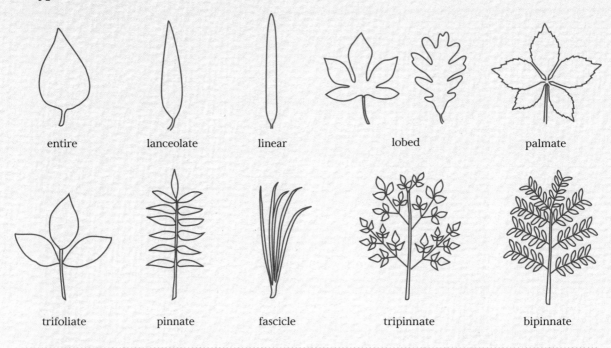

entire   lanceolate   linear   lobed   palmate

trifoliate   pinnate   fascicle   tripinnate   bipinnate

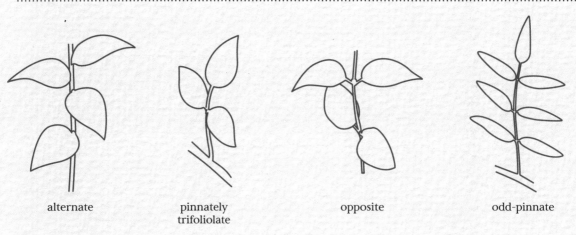

alternate   pinnately trifoliolate   opposite   odd-pinnate

Types of Inflorescence

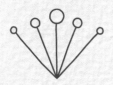

determinate

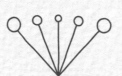

indeterminate

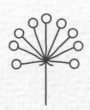

umbel
simple

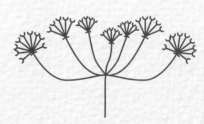

umbel
compound

APPENDIX

Quick Phonetics Guide for Some Sounds in the Squamish Language

Adapted directly from the *Squamish-English Dictionary*

Kw – qu as in *queen*

K̲w – qu as in *queen* but from farther back in the throat

K' – cu as in *cut* but sharper

K̲ – c as in *call* but farther back in the throat

Lh – similar to the thl in *athlete*

Ts – ts as in *cats*

Ts' – ts as in *cats* but sharper

U – oa as in *boat*

Uu – oa as in *boat* but longer

Xw – similar to a whispered version of wh in *what*

X̲ – a friction sound at the back of your throat

X̲w – similar to x̲ but with rounded lips

7 – glottal stop similar to in the middle of *uh-oh*

Other Incredible Plant Oils and Butters for Skincare

Cocoa butter (INCI name: *Theobroma cacao* (Cocoa) Seed Butter) is rich in antioxidants and phytochemicals, which promote blood circulation and have anti-aging properties. It can be used to treat dry skin, prevent moisture loss, and protect the skin from the sun's ultraviolet rays. Cocoa butter is also used to reduce scars, fine lines, and stretch marks. It removes rashes caused by skin conditions like eczema.

Cranberry seed oil (INCI name: *Vaccinium macrocarpon*) has a fine texture that is quickly absorbed and feels light on the skin. A little bit of cranberry seed oil goes a long way. It is suitable for all skin types and will benefit those with dry or mature skin that craves extra moisture. It is also a superior oil in body care formulations due to its unique balance of omega-3 fatty acids and naturally occurring vitamin E.

Evening primrose oil (INCI name: *Oenothera biennis*) is prized for its abundant food, health, and cosmetic uses. Evening primrose is a common wildflower found in North America, Europe, and parts of Asia. The yellow blooms only open in the evening. This particular oil should be kept refrigerated to help prolong shelf life. For cosmetic use, evening primrose oil should be added after any preparation steps that require heat.

Mango seed butter (INCI name: *Mangifera indica* seed butter) is rich in vitamins A, C, and E, and fatty acids. It moisturizes the skin and can be used to treat dry skin and other conditions like psoriasis and eczema. It also helps to soften the skin and protect it from ultraviolet damage. It rejuvenates the skin and keeps it elastic, firm, and radiant. Mango seed oil reduces inflammation on the skin, dark spots, and acne.

Meadowfoam seed oil (INCI name: *Limnanthes alba*) is an antioxidant and is rich in long-chain fatty acids. It is suitable for all skin types and can be used daily and alongside other organic skin products. It keeps the skin soft, supple, and smooth. Meadowfoam seed oil also keeps the skin moisturized, rejuvenated, and protected from damage by the sun. It reduces the appearance of acne, scars, stretch marks, wrinkles, and fine lines.

Rosehip oil (INCI name: *Rosa canina*) is considered a dry oil, meaning it absorbs quickly and doesn't leave the skin feeling oily. It is truly an amazing oil! Rosehip oil contains essential fatty acids and is a great emollient for dry or mature skin. It is also perfect for nearly any skin type and can be used in all fine skincare recipes.

Sea buckthorn oil (INCI name: *Hippophae rhamnoides*) is a very useful and highly prized oil used in skincare recipes. It can be applied directly to the skin or included within skincare preparations. This oil contains essential fatty acids, carotenes, tocopherols, and phytosterols. This is a very concentrated and nourishing oil, so I suggest using it sparingly. The oil has a deep reddish-orange hue and can stain lighter clothing. It may leave visible coloration on lighter skin tones.

Shea butter (INCI name: *Butyrospermum parkii*) contains a high concentration of fatty acids and natural vitamins. It moisturizes the skin and can also be used to treat dry, itching, peeling, and irritated skin. It reduces signs of aging, keeps the skin smooth, firm, and wrinkle-free, and restores the skin's elasticity. It is also used to heal burns, scars, and bruises, and prevents skin conditions like eczema, rashes, and dermatitis.

Additional Recipes

 ### INFUSED OIL

1 quart (1 L)
This oil can be used in the basic salve recipe on the next page.

Materials
½ cup (66–70 g) dried botanical of choice
1 quart (1 L) of oil

1 To make an infused oil, place the oil and dried botanical into the top of a double boiler. Pour water in the bottom pot, being careful not to have the water touching the bottom of the top pot.

2 Bring the water in the lower pot to a boil and then turn down to simmer.

3 Let the oil in the top of the double boiler warm gently for 2–6 hours, always checking to make sure the water in the bottom pot hasn't evaporated.

4 Let the oil cool and wipe the bottom of the top pot with a cloth to avoid any water drops coming into contact with the infused oil.

5 Strain the oil through a colander lined with cheesecloth to remove any plant materials from the infused oil.

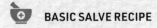 **BASIC SALVE RECIPE**

1 cup (295 g)

This recipe is great for sore muscles. I use a nettle-infused oil here, but you can use your dried botanical of choice to infuse.

Materials

1 cup (240 ml) oil (infused with plants either using the sun infusion or double boiler method; here, you can prepare ts'e<u>x</u>ts'í<u>x</u> oil from the recipe on the previous page)

¼ cup (58 g) beeswax pellets or grated beeswax, plus more if needed

2–3 drops vitamin E oil and/or rosemary oleoresin to extend shelf life

5–10 drops essential oil of your choosing (make sure they are organic and steam-distilled essential oils)

1 Pour water in the bottom pot of a double boiler, being careful not to have the water touching the bottom of the top pot. Pour the oil into the top pot. Heat the oil slowly over low heat, adding the beeswax and stirring.

2 Once the beeswax is melted, drop a few drops of the salve onto a spoon and put the spoon in the freezer for about 1 minute to test the consistency. It should be solid at room temperature. If it's still runny, add more beeswax and try the test again. Once you have the consistency you are aiming for, add the vitamin E oil, as well as the essential oils, and stir.

3 If it's ready, pour the salve into containers and let it cool thoroughly before putting the lid on. Use the salve within 1 year and make sure to label the containers with the name of the salve and the date it was created.

SAVORY DIPPING SAUCE

½ cup (120 ml)

This sauce pairs well with K̲'emeĺáý Flower Fritters (page 79).

Ingredients

2 small cloves garlic (minced and browned if preferred)

3 tablespoons light soy sauce or tamari

2 tablespoons rice vinegar

2 teaspoons sesame oil

1 Blend all the ingredients thoroughly in a blender.

2 Pour into a dipping bowl.

3 Store any unused sauce in an airtight container for up to 1 week in the refrigerator.

 BLUEBERRY AND SALAL SAUCE

½ cup (120 ml)

Serve this dipping sauce alongside Crispy Chicken Fingers with K̲wáýtsay (page 89).

Ingredients

⅓ cup (50 g) fresh blueberries

⅓ cup (50 g) fresh salal berries

2 tablespoons warm water

2 teaspoons honey

1 Place all the sauce ingredients into a blender and blend together.

2 Pour into a bowl to dip chicken fingers in.

REFERENCES

Bouchard, Randy, and Nancy J. Turner. *Ethnobotany of the Squamish Indian People of British Columbia*. Victoria, BC: British Columbia Indian Language Project, 1976.

Brach, Tara. *True Refuge: Finding Peace and Freedom in Your Own Awakened Heart*. New York: Bantam Books, 2016.

Cuerrier, Alain, Nancy J. Turner, Thiago Gomes, Ann Garibaldi, and Ashleigh Downing. "Cultural Keystone Places: Conservation and Restoration in Cultural Landscapes." *Journal of Ethnobiology* 35, no. 3 (Fall 2015): 427–448. https://doi.org/10.2993/0278-0771-35.3.427.

Deur, Douglas, and Nancy J. Turner. *Keeping It Living: Traditions of Plant Use and Cultivation on the Northwest Coast of North America*. Seattle: University of Washington Press, 2005.

Druehl, Louis D., and Bridgette Clarkston. *Pacific Seaweeds: A Guide to Common Seaweeds of the West Coast*. Pender Harbour, BC: Harbour Publishing, 2016.

Geniusz, Mary Siisip. *Plants Have So Much to Give Us, All We Have to Do is Ask: Anishinaabe Botanical Teachings*. Minneapolis: University of Minnesota Press, 2015.

Gray, Beverley. *The Boreal Herbal: Wild Food and Medicine Plants of the North*. Whitehorse, YT: Aroma Borealis Press, 2011.

Harris, James G., and Melinda Woolf Harris. *Plant Identification Terminology: An Illustrated Glossary*, 2nd Ed. Payson, UT: Spring Lake Publishing, 2009.

Hitchcock, Charles Leo, and Arthur Cronquist. Edited by David E. Giblin, Ben S. Legler, Peter F. Zika, and Richard G. Olmstead. *Flora of the Pacific Northwest: An Illustrated Manual*, 2nd Ed. Seattle: University of Washington Press, 2018.

Jacobs, Peter, and Damara Jacobs, Eds. *Sḵwx̱wú7mesh Snichim - Xwelíten Snichim: SḴEXWTS = Squamish-English Dictionary*. Seattle: University of Washington Press, 2011. Copublished with: Squamish Nation Education Department.

Joseph, Leigh. "Case Study 2: Reclaiming Our Plant Traditions: the Importance of Indigenous Foods," within "Conclusions: the Future of Ethnobotany in British Columbia," by N. J. Turner and D. Lepofsky. *BC Studies* 179 (2013): 189–209. https://ojs.library.ubc.ca/index.php/bcstudies/article/view/184543/184180.

Joseph, Leigh. "Walking on Our Lands Again: Turning to Culturally Important Plants and Indigenous Conceptualizations of Health in a Time of Cultural and Political Resurgence." *International Journal of Indigenous Health* 16, no. 1 (2021), 165–179. https://doi.org/10.32799/ijih.v16i1.33205.

Joseph, Leigh, and Nancy J. Turner. "'The Old Foods Are the New Foods!': Erosion and Revitalization of Indigenous Food Systems in Northwestern North America." *Frontiers in Sustainable Food Systems* 4, 270 (2020). DOI:10.3389/fsufs.2020.596237.

Kimmerer, Robin Wall. *Braiding Sweetgrass: Indigenous Wisdom, Scientific Knowledge and the Teachings of Plants*. Minneapolis, MN: Milkweed Editions, 2013.

Klinkenberg, Brian, Ed. *E-Flora BC: Electronic Atlas of the Flora of British Columbia*. Lab for Advanced Spatial Analysis, Department of Geography, University of British Columbia, Vancouver, 2021. Accessed March 1, 2022. https://ibis.geog.ubc.ca/biodiversity/eflora/.

Lotioncrafter. Accessed April 5, 2022. https://lotioncrafter.com.

MacKinnon, Andy, Jim Pojar, and Ray Coupe. *Plants of Northern British Columbia*, 2nd Ed. Tukwila, WA: Lone Pine Publishing, 2021.

Maracle, Lee. *My Conversations with Canadians*. Toronto: Book*hug Press, 2017.

Matthews, Major James Skitt. *Conversations with Khahtsahlano, 1932–1954*. Vancouver: City Hall Press, 1955.

Miskelly, Kristen, and James Miskelly. "Why Native Plants?" *Satinflower Nurseries*. Accessed March 10, 2022. https://satinflower.ca/pages/about-native-plants.

Mountain Rose Herbs. Accessed April 5, 2022. https://mountainroseherbs.com.

New Directions Aromatics. Accessed April 2, 2022. https://www.newdirectionsaromatics.ca.

Pojar, Jim, and Andy MacKinnon. *Plants of the Pacific Northwest Coast: Washington, Oregon, British Columbia & Alaska.* Vancouver: BC Ministry of Forests; Tukwila, WA: Lone Pine Publishing, 1994.

Shakespeare, William. *Romeo and Juliet.* Blount and Jaggard: 1623.

Simard, Suzanne. *Finding the Mother Tree: Uncovering the Wisdom and Intelligence of the Forest.* New York: Penguin Random House, 2022.

Simpson, Leanne Betasamosake. *As We've Always Done: Indigenous Freedom Through Radical Resistance.* Minneapolis: University of Minnesota Press, 2017.

Thayer, Samuel. *The Forager's Harvest: A Guide to Identifying, Harvesting, and Preparing Edible Wild Plants.* Weyerhaeuser, WI: Forager's Harvest Press, 2006.

Turner, Nancy J. *Ancient Pathways, Ancestral Knowledge: Ethnobotany and Ecological Wisdom of Indigenous Peoples of Northwestern North America, Volume 1.* Montreal: McGill–Queen's University Press, 2014.

Turner, Nancy J. *Food Plants of Coastal First Peoples.* Vancouver: UBC Press, 1995.

Turner, Nancy J. *The Earth's Blanket: Traditional Teachings for Sustainable Living.* Vancouver: Douglas & McIntyre, 2005.

Turner, Nancy J., and Patrick von Aderkas. *The North American Guide to Common Poisonous Plants and Mushrooms.* Portland: Timber Press, 2009.

Turner, Nancy J., and Richard Joseph Hebda. *Saanich Ethnobotany: Culturally Important Plants of the WSANEC People.* Victoria, BC: Royal BC Museum, 2014.

Vitt, Dale Hadley, J. Marsh, and R. Bovey. *Mosses, Lichens and Ferns of Northwest North America: A Photographic Field Guide.* Tukwila, WA: Lone Pine Publishing, 1988.

ACKNOWLEDGMENTS

I wish to acknowledge my Squamish ancestors who carried with them the knowledge of the land and plants for future generations to learn from. I wish to thank the plants that I work with and the landscape on which they grow for nourishing our Skwxwú7mesh People for thousands of years.

I want to thank my children, Ava and Jake Glazier, and my husband, Lee Glazier, for being so supportive of me and the work I do, and for the endless hours out harvesting together on the land.

Thanks to my grandparents, Rose and Larry Joseph on my father's side and Duna and Bert Levy on my mother's side, and to my great-uncle Chester and great-aunt Eva for creating my childhood experiences of being on the land and sharing nourishing meals together in their home on the Nanaimo River.

I wish to thank my father, Chief Floyd Joseph, for teaching me from an early age how to sit with elders and listen to and absorb their teachings, and for helping me to foster a love for nature and for our Skwxwú7mesh culture.

Thank you to my mother, Eve Joseph, for teaching me how to walk in the world with an open mind and heart, how to approach expressing myself creatively, and also for the hours of editing she and my stepfather Patrick Friesen have put into my writing career so far!

Thank you to my siblings, Saul and Salia Joseph, for their support, love, and laughter. I admire you both so much.

Thank you to my auntie Joy Joseph-McCullough, who has been my mentor and teacher and has guided me into community here in Squamish.

Thank you to Chum for all the times spent along the trails teaching me about our plant medicines and my responsibility to share the knowledge I gain with our Skwxwú7mesh youth.

Thank you to the late Kwaxsistalla, Adam Dick, and his partner, Kim Recalma-Clutesi, for all the wonderful times spent on the land learning.

I want to thank my dear friend and colleague Dr. Nancy Turner for the years of teaching and mentorship and for the respect and love that she brings to her work.

Thank you to Myia Antone and Sarah Jeffreys for translating the Sḵwx̱wú7mesh language and contributing the pronunciation of the Sḵwx̱wú7mesh words.

Thank you to Jim Pojar for bringing an expert eye to the editing of the plant profiles. It is a pleasure to work with you.

Thank you to Sharon Brown and Andreas Schroeder for opening your lovely writing cabin to me.

To Rachel Dickens and Adam Hart, thanks for your support on the recipe development and writing process.

Finally, thank you to the team from Quarto Publishing, my editors Katie Moore and Elizabeth You, for all the support in helping me bring this book from a dream into reality.

ABOUT THE AUTHOR

Leigh Joseph (ancestral name Styawat) is an ethnobotanist (a plant scientist who studies the interrelationships between people and plants), community-based researcher, and entrepreneur from the Squamish First Nation. She contributes to cultural knowledge renewal in connection to Indigenous plant- and land-based relationships and provides an Indigenous lens to her field of study.

Leigh's research examines the link between healing and the renewal of Indigenous plant knowledge and practices related to ethnobotany, and is influenced by her experience as an Indigenous woman reconnecting to her cultural roots. Wherever possible, she draws on ancestral teachings that are connected to traditional plants and the land in her research.

Leigh began creating skincare products as a creative outlet for her research and to use for her children, crafting them with plant ingredients she sustainably harvested. She gave some early iterations of products as gifts to elders and had a very positive response, which led her to start a skincare business.

As founder of Sḵwálwen Botanicals (https://skwalwen.com), Leigh brings together Indigenous science and self-care, providing gentle and effective skincare products that draw from the ceremonial aspects of plants. Incorporating sustainably harvested and sourced botanicals, Sḵwálwen unites ancestral traditions with modern beauty rituals, empowering people to connect to themselves and the natural world.

Through its philanthropic partnerships, Sḵwálwen elevates Indigenous communities and shines a light on the strength and resilience of Indigenous Peoples.

ABOUT THE RECIPE CONTRIBUTORS

Rachel Dickens is from Lax Kxeen in Prince Rupert and is a member of the Ts'msyen Nation Lax Kw'alaams. She is a registered Dietitian (RD), Certified Diabetes Educator (CDE), and PhD student.

Adam Hart, having healed his own health with the help of plant nutrition, now shares his journey with others as a Holistic Mindset Coach and a national bestselling cookbook author.

INDEX